Roberto Patarca-Montero, MD, PhD

Chronic Fatigue Syndrome and the Body's Immune Defense System

Pre-publication
REVIEWS,
COMMENTARIES,
EVALUATIONS . . .

"*Chronic Fatigue Syndrome and the Body's Immune Defense System* is a comprehensive and concise selection of pertinent research from the world's CFS literature. The standard of scholarship and unbiased presentations will be welcomed by physicians and others interested in the latest etiology concepts and resulting therapeutic interventions. Wherever CFS is treated, this excellent treatise and reference section should be available."

Dr. R. Bruce Duncan, FRCS, FRACS
Director,
Virutherapy Clinic,
Wellington, New Zealand

"This is an incredible book. It brings together a wealth of information that has been generated by researchers around the world during the past twenty years. It is possibly the first major book to concentrate, in an in-depth manner, on the immunological anomalies in CFS patients. This publication contains an encyclopedic amount of immunological information useful to the physician, researcher, or informed patient who wishes to acquire a better knowledge of CFS. It will remain an important adjunct to our understanding of these complex disease processes that constitute the CFS spectrum of diseases. This is a necessary reference publication for any author who contemplates publishing a research paper or book on CFS. The references included are worth the price of the book.

The author comes with superb credentials. He is Director of Clinical Immunology at the University of Miami School of Medicine, perhaps the foremost American center known for its most continuous and resolute investigation of immune anomalies in CFS."

Byron Hyde, MD
Chairman,
Nightingale Research Foundation,
Ottawa, Canada

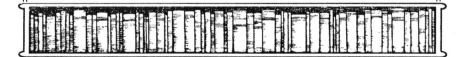

More pre-publication
REVIEWS, COMMENTARIES, EVALUATIONS . . .

"This book is an excellent scientific companion to *Concise Encyclopedia of Chronic Fatigue Syndrome,* which has already been published by the same author. The latter gives an excellent résumé of the multifarious clinical findings on this illness, and the present book gives a superb account of the research into the complex histological changes and abnormalities that simultaneously occur. This book is thus a synthesis of the reports by several hundred medical research experts based on worldwide studies.

The detailed information relating to the autoimmune consequences that were alluded to in the former book is here. It is developed in exceptional depth as a result of these studies into the large array of varying responses at the complex cellular levels that comprise the autoimmune system."

Dr. John Richardson, M B, BS
Research Founder Member,
Newcastle Research Group,
United Kingdom;
Author, *Enteroviral and Toxin Mediated ME/CFS and Other Organ Pathologies*

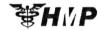

The Haworth Medical Press®
An Imprint of The Haworth Press, Inc.
New York   London   Oxford

Chronic Fatigue Syndrome and the Body's Immune Defense System

THE HAWORTH MEDICAL PRESS®
Haworth Research Series
on Malaise, Fatigue, and Debilitation

Roberto Patarca-Montero, MD, PhD
Senior Editor

Concise Encyclopedia of Chronic Fatigue Syndrome by Roberto Patarca-Montero

CFIDS, Fibromyalgia, and the Virus-Allergy Link: Hidden Viruses, Allergies, and Uncommon Fatigue/Pain Disorders by R. Bruce Duncan

Adolescence and Myalgic Encephalomyelitis/Chronic Fatigue Syndrome: Journeys with the Dragon by Naida Edgar Brotherston

Phytotherapy of Chronic Fatigue Syndrome: Evidence-Based and Potentially Useful Botanicals in the Treatment of CFS by Roberto Patarca-Montero

Autogenic Training: A Mind-Body Approach to the Treatment of Fibromyalgia and Chronic Pain Syndrome by Micah R. Sadigh

Enteroviral and Toxin Mediated Myalgic Encephalomyelitis/Chronic Fatigue Syndrome and Other Organ Pathologies by John Richardson

Treatment of Chronic Fatigue Syndrome in the Antiviral Revolution Era by Roberto Patarca-Montero

Chronic Fatigue Syndrome, Christianity, and Culture: Between God and an Illness by James M. Rotholz

The Concise Encyclopedia of Fibromyalgia and Myofascial Pain by Roberto Patarca-Montero

Chronic Fatigue Syndrome and the Body's Immune Defense System by Roberto Patarca-Montero

Chronic Fatigue Syndrome, Genes, and Infection: The ETA-1/OP Paradigm by Roberto Patarca-Montero

Chronic Fatigue Syndrome and the Body's Immune Defense System

Roberto Patarca-Montero, MD, PhD

The Haworth Medical Press®
An Imprint of The Haworth Press, Inc.
New York • London • Oxford

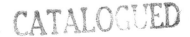

Published by

The Haworth Medical Press®, an imprint of The Haworth Press, Inc., 10 Alice Street, Binghamton, NY 13904-1580.

Medicine is an ever-changing science. As new research and clinical experience broaden our knowledge, changes in treatment and drug therapy are required. While many suggestions for drug usages are made herein, the book is intended for educational purposes only, and the author, editor, and publisher do not accept liability in the event of negative consequences incurred as a result of information presented in this book. We do not claim that this information is necessarily accurate by the rigid, scientific standard applied for medical proof, and therefore make no warranty, expressed or implied, with respect to the material herein contained. Therefore the patient is urged to check the product information sheet included in the package of each drug he or she plans to administer to be certain the protocol followed is not in conflict with the manufacturer's inserts. When a discrepancy arises between these inserts and information in this book, the physician is encouraged to use his or her best professional judgment.

The author has exhaustively researched all available sources to ensure the accuracy and completeness of the information contained in this book. The publisher and author assume no responsibility for errors, inaccuracies, omissions, or any inconsistency herein.

Cover design by Marylouise E. Doyle.

Library of Congress Cataloging-in-Publication Data

Patarca-Montero, Roberto.
    Chronic fatigue syndrome and the body's immune defense system / Roberto Patarca-Montero.
       p. cm.
    Includes bibliographical references and index.
    ISBN 0-7890-1529-3 (hard : alk. paper)—ISBN 0-7890-1530-7 (soft : alk. paper)
    1. Chronic fatigue syndrome. 2. Immunity. I. Title.
    [DNLM: 1. Fatigue Syndrome, Chronic—immunology. 2. Immune System. WB 146 P294c 2001]
RB150.F37 P377 2001
616'.0478—dc21
                                                2001051688

CONTENTS

**Chapter 1. Overview of the Human Immune System
and Its Relevance to Chronic Fatigue Syndrome**　　　**1**

**Chapter 2. Cross-Talk Between the Immune, Endocrine,
and Nervous Systems**　　　**7**

Neuroendocrinology of Chronic Fatigue Syndrome　　　14

**Chapter 3. The Soldiers of the Immune Army:
Immune Cell Phenotypic Distributions**　　　**21**

T Lymphocytes　　　22
B Lymphocytes　　　26
Natural Killer Cells　　　26
Neutrophils　　　26

Chapter 4. Immune Cell Function　　　**27**

T and B Lymphocytes　　　27
Natural Killer Cells　　　29
Monocytes　　　32
Eosinophils　　　32

**Chapter 5. Cytokines and Other Soluble
Immune Mediators**　　　**35**

Cytokines　　　36
Immunoglobulins　　　45
Autoantibodies　　　46
Circulating Immune Complexes　　　47

**Chapter 6. Potential Infectious and Autoimmune
Etiologies for Chronic Fatigue Syndrome**　　　**49**

Infectious Agents As Possible Direct Causes of CFS　　　49
Autoimmunity and CFS: Infectious Agents As Possible
　Indirect Causes of CFS　　　56

Chapter 7. The Th1/Th2 Imbalance Paradigm in Chronic Fatigue Syndrome   **61**

Chapter 8. Immunotherapy of Chronic Fatigue Syndrome: Th1/Th2 Balance Modulation   **69**

Lymph Node Cell-Based Immunotherapy   71
Mycobacterium Vaccae   73
Staphylococcal Vaccine   75
Sizofiran   76
Panax Ginseng   77
Juzen-Taiho-To   78

Chapter 9. Concluding Remarks   **79**

References   **81**

Index   **115**

ABOUT THE AUTHOR

Roberto Patarca-Montero, MD, PhD, HCLD, is Assistant Professor of Medicine, Microbiology, and Immunology and also serves as Research Director of the E. M. Papper Laboratory of Clinical Immunology at the University of Miami School of Medicine. Previously, he was Assistant Professor of Pathology at the Dana-Farber Cancer Institute and Harvard Medical School in Boston. Dr. Patarca serves as editor of *Critical Reviews in Oncogenesis* and the *Journal of Chronic Fatigue Syndrome.* He is also the author or co-author of more than 100 articles in journals or books, as well as the *Concise Encyclopedia of Chronic Fatigue Syndrome* and *Chronic Fatigue Syndrome: Advances in Epidemiologic, Clinical, and Basic Science Research* (The Haworth Press). He is currently conducting research on immunotherapy of AIDS and chronic fatigue syndrome. Dr. Patarca is a member of the Board of Directors of the American Association for Chronic Fatigue Syndrome and the Acquired Non-HIV Immune Diseases Foundation.

Chapter 1

Overview of the Human Immune System and Its Relevance to Chronic Fatigue Syndrome

The human body is made up of particular groups of cells, each performing specialized functions. Those of the immune system, which circulate in the blood (white blood cells) or populate many tissues and mucous surfaces, and predominate in certain organs (such as the spleen and bone marrow), act as an army in charge of defending the body by attacking foreign invaders and cancer cells, and disposing of the remains of dead cells. The immune system cells closely network with each other and with cells of other bodily systems through both direct interactions or a series of message conveyors known as cytokines ("cyto" stands for cell, and "kines" for movers, i.e., messages that get cells going), which are endowed with the capacity to interact with different cell types and modulate their function. For instance, macrophages (from the greek word for "big eaters"), immune cells that survey the body for the presence of microbes or dead cells, engulf these particles, digest them, and present the resulting pieces to the T cells (or T lymphocytes), the generals of the immune system army. The T cells (the "T" comes from the observation that they were originally found to predominate in the thymus) then decide if the digested particle pieces are foreign to the body or abnormal. If T cells are presented with a foreign or abnormal particle, they become activated, i.e., they start to divide and secrete cytokines to stimulate other T cells, macrophages/monocytes, natural killer cells (immune cells that are able to kill microbial infected or cancer cells by themselves, with or without orders from the generals), or B cells (cells that act similar to cannons that fire the bullets known as immunoglobulins) (the "B" comes from the observation that they are the predominant cells in the bursa of birds).

Some of the cytokines produced in the immunological battlefield travel into the protected environment of the central nervous system and warn the brain that the body is defending itself from a foreign invader. One such cytokine is interleukin-1 ("inter" meaning between and "leukin" referring to leucocyte or white blood cell, because cytokines were originally believed to be message conveyors only between white blood cells). Interleukin-1 (abbreviated IL-1) travels to the region of the brain known as the hypothalamus and affects the body's thermostat, a process that leads to fever (microbes usually replicate less efficiently at higher body temperatures) and somnolence (sleep allows the body to spare and focus energy on the battle against the invading microbe). Other cytokines, such as tumor necrosis factor, are also fever inducers, the so-called pyrogens.

The immune army activation process is mediated by the group of T-cell generals known as T-helper cells, which derive their name from the fact that they "help" or "boost" the immune attack. Another group of T-cell generals, known as the T-suppressor cells, is in charge of quenching the immune response and returning the army to its resting state. As in the army, where one can identify the rank and function of soldiers or officers by their uniform and insignia, the cells of the immune system carry particular surface markers that are associated with particular functions and have been given cluster designation or cluster differentiation (CD) numbers. All T cells carry the CD3 surface marker, also known as the T-cell receptor, the portal of presentation of particles to T cells by macrophages/monocytes and B cells, the so-called antigen-presenting cells. T-helper cells carry on their surface a molecule known as CD4, and T-suppressor cells carry CD8. T-helper cells are further subclassified into two types. T-helper type 1 (Th1) cells produce a group of cytokines that predominantly stimulate macrophages/monocytes and natural killer cells, the cells best suited to directly attack microbes that hide and replicate in the cells. The type of immune response favored by Th1 cells is therefore called cellular immunity. T-helper type 2 (Th2) cells preferentially stimulate the function of B cells and the production of antibodies. This so-called humoral immunity is best suited to deal with parasites that are too large to be killed by individual macrophages/monocytes or natural killer cells and need to be coated first with the immunoglobulin bullets to then be attacked by other proteins in the blood, such as complement, or by the other cells of the immune army. Undifferentiated T-helper cells that are neither Th1 nor Th2 are designated Th0.

The two types of T-helper cell responses were first documented in mice. Some strains of mice differentially succumbed to particular infections based on the type of T-helper response that was predominant in that particular strain (inbreeding of mice strains allowed the selection of strains that would predominantly respond with either a Th1 or a Th2 response). Although in humans the dichotomy in T-helper cell responses is not as clear-cut, the Th1/Th2 paradigm is still valid. Human T-helper cell responses have either a Th1- or Th2-type bias and certain disease states can be associated with a predominance of one or the other T-helper cell type response. For instance, disease progression in acquired immunodeficiency syndrome (AIDS) is associated with a shift from a Th1-type predominance to a more undifferentiated Th0-type response. The AIDS virus also replicates more readily in Th2- and Th0-type cells. Based on these observations, several therapeutic interventions for AIDS are aimed at favoring a shift back toward a Th1-type response. Some cytokines, such as interleukin-2 (IL-2) and interleukin-12 (IL-12), have the ability of favoring such a shift but their direct administration to humans, particularly IL-12, is associated with toxicities. Administration of IL-2, a strong stimulator of natural killer cells, is used as a therapeutic modality in the treatment of patients with certain neoplasias, such as renal cell carcinoma and melanoma.

Other diseases are associated with a predominance of a Th2-type response. As a metaphor of many occasions in human history, the policing and military roles of the bodily army can turn against the body that it is supposed to protect. In these situations, normal components of the body start being recognized as foreign, and diseases, collectively known as autoimmune diseases, ensue. Systemic lupus erythematosus and rheumatoid arthritis are examples of autoimmune diseases, which are characterized by the stimulation of B cells to produce antibody bullets that attack certain tissues in the body and produce a sequela of destruction. The predominant type of T-helper cell generals that are involved in autoimmune diseases are T-helper type 2 cells. The same is true for allergic reactions and for asthma, which are associated with increased production of one type of immunoglobulin bullets, the E type, in response to environmental factors that are innocuous to most individuals.

Although chronic fatigue syndrome (CFS) is an ailment of yet unknown etiology, it is characterized in at least one-third of patients, mostly among those with an acute onset, i.e., following a flulike illness, by evidence of activation of the immune army, an observation which lends support to the hypothesis that CFS is caused by an infection that either lingers chronically or leaves an autoimmune sequela. In this respect, it is known that microbes can cause damage either directly or indirectly. As they attack a microbe, some microbial components may resemble human components, and the body may end up generating antibody bullets that can also recognize bodily components, a process termed *molecular mimicry* that can lead to autoimmune disease manifestations. The latter process is also favored by genetic predisposition in the form of particular variants of the human leukocyte antigen (HLA) molecules, the proteins that antigen-presenting cells use to present particles to the T cells.

It is curious that although the immune army is activated in a subset of CFS patients, the soldiers of the immune army, particularly the T cells and natural killer cells, function poorly. T cells from CFS patients have a decreased capacity to divide and generate new T cells, and the natural killer cells have significantly decreased "killing" or cytotoxic activity. In CFS, not only is the function of the T cells impaired but the repertoire of T-helper cells is also biased, as in autoimmune diseases, toward a Th2-type response. Activated T-helper cell generals from CFS patients produce less interferon-gamma, a Th1-type cytokine, and more interleukin-5, a Th2-type cytokine. These features combined create a pervasive immunological battlefield-like environment in CFS patients that is Th2-type predominant with compromised cellular immunity and ability of the body to deal with microbes along with the presence of auto antibodies. The triggers and maintenance factors of the Th2-type predominance are unknown but could include infections, toxins, prior immunizations, hormonal status changes, or a combination thereof.

Based on these observations, several therapeutic interventions being tested are aimed at favoring a shift of the T-helper cell responses of CFS patients from a Th2- to a Th1-type predominant pattern. These approaches are based on the use of *Staphylococcus* vaccine, influenza and/or rubella virus vaccines, *Mycobacterium vaccae* vaccine, poly I-C, and autologous reinfusion of lymph node cells that had been expanded and activated outside the body with Th1-type inducing cytokines, such as interleukin-2. Some of these therapeutic interventions are based on the old medical wisdom of curing one infection by giving another to the patient, and most appear in published patents. These immunotherapies have shown promising results with clinical improvement as assessed by functional status and cognitive measures. Some other interventions are based on the use of herbal products, such as *Panax ginseng,* which have been associated with improved Th1-type responses. Further studies will allow us to elucidate the factors that mediate Th-2 response predominance in CFS, as well as the association of particular cytokines with different CFS symptoms. The following chapters will further detail our knowledge and experience with the immunological correlates of chronic fatigue syndrome.

Chapter 2

Cross-Talk Between the Immune, Endocrine, and Nervous Systems

The nervous and immune systems respond to internal and external challenges and communicate and regulate each other by means of shared or system-unique hormones, growth factors, neurotransmitters, and neuromodulators. Therefore, the nervous and immune systems are two major adaptive systems of the body. During an immune response, the nervous and immune systems communicate with each other, and this process is important to maintain homeostasis or balanced physiological function. The hypothalamic-pituitary-adrenal (HPA) axis and the sympathetic nervous system are two of the major systems involved in the cross-talk between the nervous and immune systems (Elenkov et al., 2000).

Elenkov et al. (2000) point out that evidence accumulated over the past twenty years suggests that norepinephrine (NE) fulfills the criteria for neurotransmitter/neuromodulator in lymphoid organs. Primary and secondary lymphoid organs receive extensive sympathetic/ noradrenergic innervation. Under stimulation, NE is released from the sympathetic nerve terminals in these organs, and the target immune cells express adrenoreceptors. Through stimulation of these receptors, locally released NE, or circulating cathecolamines such as epinephrine, affect lymphocyte traffic, circulation, and proliferation, and modulate cytokine production and the functional activity of different lymphoid cells. NE and epinephrine, through stimulation of the β2-adrenoreceptor-cAMP-protein kinase A pathway, inhibit the production of type 1/proinflammatory cytokines, such as interleukin-12, tumor necrosis factor-alpha, and interferon-gamma by antigen-presenting cells and T-helper (Th)1 cells, whereas they stimulate the production of type 2/anti-inflammatory cytokines, such as IL-10 and transforming growth factor-beta. Through this mechanism, endogenous catecholamines may cause a systemic selective suppression of

Th1 responses and cellular immunity, and a shift toward a Th2 cytokine profile and predominance of humoral immunity. On the other hand, in certain local responses, and under certain conditions, catecholamines may actually boost regional immune responses through induction of IL-1, tumor necrosis factor-alpha, and primarily IL-8 production. Thus, the activation of the sympathetic nervous system during an immune response might be aimed to localize the inflammatory response, through induction of neutrophil accumulation and stimulation of more specific humoral immune responses, although systematically it may suppress Th1 responses and thus protect the organism from the detrimental effects of proinflammatory cytokines and other products of activated macrophages (Elenkov et al., 2000).

Further evidence for the interconnections between the nervous and immune systems comes from studies of stress. Similar alterations in central catecholamine neurotransmitter levels are associated with immune activity and stressor exposure, alterations that are more pronounced in aged as opposed to younger animals (Shanks et al., 1994). For example, a decreased norepinephrine turnover in the hypothalami and brainstem of rats occurs at the peak of the immune response to sheep red blood cells (Besedovsky et al., 1983; Vasina et al., 1975), and increased serotonin metabolism is associated with depressed Arthus reaction and plaque-forming cell response in rats stressed either by overcrowding lasting two weeks or more or by repeated immobilization for four days (Boranic, 1990; Boranic et al., 1982). The long-term effects of these acute changes are evidenced by chronic variable stress, which facilitates tumor growth (Basso et al., 1992) and is associated with immune dysregulation in multiple sclerosis (Foley et al., 1992). The HPA axis plays a pivotal role in stress-mediated changes, and stimulation of corticotropin-releasing factor in the central nervous system (De Souza, 1993; Irwin, 1993) has been shown to suppress rapidly a variety of immune responses, an effect that can be blocked by infusion into the brain of alpha-melanocyte-stimulating hormone, a tridecapeptide derived from pro-opiomelanocortin (Weiss et al., 1994).

Besides external stimuli, intrinsic imbalances in neurotransmitter levels affect the immune system either directly by acting on immunocompetent cells or indirectly via induction of hormonal secretions. For instance, depression is associated with neurotransmitter imbalances and with decreased natural killer cell cytotoxic activity (Hebert and Cohen, 1993; Irwin, Caldwell, et al., 1990; Irwin, Patterson, et al., 1990; Schleifer et al., 1989). Moreover, several studies have documented the existence of striking physiologic, neuroendocrine, metabolic, and pharmacologic differences between depressed and normal subjects and between depressed and severely ill subjects (Lechin, van der Dijs, Acosta, et al., 1983; Lechin, van der Dijs, Gomez, et al., 1983; Lechin et al., 1985, 1987, 1989, 1994). Major depression is accompanied by an increased production of IL-1beta and IL-1 receptor antagonist (IL-1Ra) (Maes et al., 1995). In depressed subjects, there was a significant and positive relationship between serum IL-1Ra levels and severity of illness, but no significant relationships with markers of HPA-axis activity (Maes et al., 1995). An eight-week stress exposure induced an increase in the ability of splenocytes from Wistar rats to produce IL-1 and IL-2 and to proliferate after stimulation with concanavalin A, activities that were reversed by the antidepressant effects of imipramine administration but not by imipramine alone (Kubera et al., 1996).

The examples previously mentioned illustrate the fact that disorders, or persistent noxious stimulation, of the neuroimmunological circuitry can lead to, or result from, neurological, immunological, psychiatric, or multiorgan pathology. The latter link has encouraged a search for neuroimmunological markers with functional or pathological correlates in many disease states. In this respect, the immune system and several endocrine axes communicate with each other through a network of molecules that collectively produce a coordinated response to immune challenges. This phenomenon, which is necessary for the survival of the organism, is thought to involve the release, by activated cells in the periphery, of proteins, called cytokines, which inform the brain about immune activation. The brain then organizes a series of neuroendocrine responses that participate in the regulation of the host response. Cytokines produce HPA-axis activation in response to various threats to homeostasis (Turnbull and Rivier, 1995a,b). The extensive interactions between different cytokines, the broad spectrum of pathophysiologies associated with increased cytokine production, and the number of tissues/cells capable of either synthesizing or responding to cytokines, suggest that multiple mechanisms mediate the influence of cytokines on the HPA axis.

IL-1 is the most potent cytokine in the activation of the HPA axis during infection and therefore leads to an increase in glucocoticoid levels. In turn, glucocorticoids, in a feedback loop, inhibit the production of IL-1 induced by endotoxin (Paez Pereda et al., 1996). Acute activation of the pituitary-adrenal axis of rats by administration of cytokines (at least IL-1, IL-6, and TNF) in vivo is not mediated by a direct action of these cytokines at the level of the pituitary and/or adrenal gland (van der Meer, Hermus, et al., 1996; van der Meer, Sweep, et al., 1996). Hypothalamic IL-1alpha, IL-1beta, and IL-6 mRNA levels may be involved in the antipyretic effects of a pretreatment with high doses of corticosterone, effects that are rapidly reversible (Chai et al., 1996). IL-1alpha, IL-1beta, IL-2, IL-6, and TNF-alpha can also affect cell motility, bacterial phagocytosis, induction of nitric oxide synthase, and the release of biogenic amines by molluscan hemocytes. Moreover, the latter cytokines can bind to and compete with corticotropin-releasing factor for the same membrane hemocyte receptor, an observation that indicates that these molecules are ancestral and have maintained their pleiotropicity, functional redundancy, and receptor promiscuity (Ottaviani and Franchini, 1995). The inflammation mediators prostaglandins (PG), especially PGE2, play a significant role in mediating corticotropin-releasing hormone and ACTH secretion by IL-1. Circulating PGE2 is not involved in the ACTH response to intravenous administration of IL-1beta, an observation which indicates that the site of action of PGE2 mediating the hormonal response is most likely in the brain (Watanobe et al., 1995).

Intracerebroventricular infusion of rats with IL-1beta induced significant increases in plasma adrenocorticotropin (ACTH) and corticosterone levels. Immunoneutralization of corticotropin-releasing hormone (CRH) significantly decreased, and macrophage depletion significantly increased, the stimulation of the hypothalamus-pituitary axis by IL-1. Administration of high doses of dexamethasone completely abolished the stimulation of the HPA axis by IL-1beta, an observation that fits well with the concept of an immunoregulatory feedback between IL-1beta and glucocorticoids (van der Meer, Hermus, et al., 1996; van der Meer, Sweep, et al., 1996). Stress down-regulates lipopolysaccharide-induced expression of proinflammatory cytokines (IL-1alpha, IL-1Ra, IL-6, and TNF-alpha) in the spleen, pituitary, and brain of mice (Goujon, Parnet, Cremona, et al., 1995; Goujon, Parnet, Laye, et al., 1995), an effect that is likely mediated by glucocorticoids. Ether-laparatomy stress in mice results in a selective increase in pituitary IL-1 receptors and a significant decrease in pituitary receptors for corticotropin-releasing factor, a major regulator of the endocrine response to stress (Takao et al., 1995, 1996).

Intravenous administration of IL-1beta induces a significantly higher ACTH response in female than in male rats, and this sexual difference is abolished by gonadectomy in both sexes. By contrast, ACTH secretion after immobilization stress, a nonimmunological stressor, is statistically the same in males and females, but tended to be higher in gonadectomized males than in gonadectomized females. These results may suggest a dissociative regulation by gonadal steroids of IL-1beta-induced and immobilization-induced ACTH responses in the rat. The sexual difference in ACTH response to IL-1beta may represent another example of the sexually dismorphic immunological activity, which is known to be higher in females than in males (Watanobe et al., 1996).

Although IL-1beta inhibits the gonadotropin-supported accumulation of progesterone, ovarian granulosa cells secrete a factor with IL-1-like activity that does not affect the basal or follicle-stimulating hormone (FSH)-stimulated accumulation of progesterone (Kokia et al., 1995). IL-1alpha directly inhibits the production of estradiol by human ovarian granulosa cells. IL-1alpha and IL-1beta also exert indirect effects on steroid production via white blood cells that are usually present in granulosa cell cultures (Best and Hill, 1995). Testicular macrophages have a reduced ability to secrete bioactive IL-1, an observation that is consistent with an altered capacity for immune responses within the testis (Hayes et al., 1996).

With regard to the influence of cytokines on the hypothalamic-pituitary-gonadal axis, we know that the injection of these proteins lowers gonadotropin-releasing hormone release, which in turn inhibits luteinizing hormone (LH) secretion. These changes would be expected to decrease sex steroid production and, indeed, estrogens and testosterone are low in female and male rats, respectively, following intracerebroventricular (ICV) injection of IL-1beta. There is, however, another possibility that central cytokines could alter ovarian and testicular function independently of changes in gonadotropin levels. Prolonged ICV infusion of the cytokine into the female rat brain produced a dramatic rise in progesterone levels. The absence of a comparable change in the progesterone release of males infused with IL-1beta, and the presence of marked surges of prolactin in the females, suggests that IL-1beta altered ovarian function, and that the persistence of large corpora lutea-induced prolactin (PRL) release. The possibility that the cytokine might stimulate the brain circuits that regulate PRL release, although possible, appears remote, because male rats injected with IL-1beta showed significantly blunted PRL levels. In intact adult male rats, ICV IL-1beta administration caused the expected decrease in LH and testosterone levels, but was also accompanied by a loss of testicular responsiveness to gonadotropins. Although elevated levels of corticosteroids are known to interfere with normal gonadal steroidogenesis, blockade of IL-1-induced corticosterone release did not reverse the inhibitory influence of the cytokine. One mechanism that deserves attention is the possibility that ICV injection of IL-1beta might increase circulating cytokine levels, and indeed plasma IL-6 concentrations were significantly elevated in rats treated with IL-1beta. This humoral mechanism may disrupt testicular function through the documented inhibitory effects of bloodborne cytokines on Leydig cell function. In addition, brain cytokines might influence a variety of peripheral events through direct, possibly neural, connections (Turnbull and Rivier, 1995a,b). The effects of anabolic steroids also illustrate the interaction between the immune, nervous, and endocrine systems. The deleterious effects of anabolic steroid use include sterility, gynecomastia in males, acne, balding, psychological changes, and increased risks of heart disease and liver neoplasia. Both 17-beta and 17-alpha esterified anabolic steroids directly induce the production of the inflammatory cytokines IL-1beta and TNF-alpha from human peripheral blood lymphocytes, but had no effect on IL-2 or IL-10 production (Hughes et al., 1995).

The neurotoxic effects of cytokines, and perhaps indirectly bacterial endotoxins, could be mediated by the stimulation of immunocompetent cells in the brain to produce toxic concentrations of nitric oxide (NO) and reactive nitrogen oxides. Nitric oxide is a short-lived, diffusible molecule that has a variety of biological activities including vaso-relaxation, neurotransmission, and cytotoxicity. Both constitutive and inducible NO synthases have been described in astrocytes in vivo, and newborn mouse cortical astrocytes, when coincubated with neonatal mouse cerebellar granule cells or hippocampal neurons, induce nitric oxide-mediated neurotoxicity upon stimulation with either endotoxin or TNF-alpha and IL-1beta. Meningeal fibroblasts treated with TNF-alpha display nitric oxide-mediated neurotoxic activity on granule cells (Skaper et al., 1995). IL-1Ra and soluble TNF-receptor (sTNF-R) do not significantly reduce the meningeal inflammatory response associated with intracisternal inoculation of *Hemophilus influenzae* type b lipooligosaccharide, and therefore may not be used to treat this infectious condition (Paris et al., 1995). Thalidomide, on the other hand, inhibits TNF-alpha, but not IL-1, release into the cerebrospinal fluid (CSF) in models of rabbit bacterial meningitis (Burroughs et al., 1995). IL-1 and TNF-alpha levels are elevated in brain tissue of individuals who died of AIDS, and TNF-alpha levels correlate with the severity of AIDS dementia complex. The latter cytokine likely stimulates reactive astrocytosis and nitric oxide production (Vitkovic et al., 1995; Chao et al., 1995; Lee et al., 1995). Agents that suppress nitric oxide production or inhibit N-methyl-D-aspartate receptors may protect against neuronal damage in cytokine-induced neurodegenerative disorders.

All of the previous examples of the interconnectivity between different bodily systems is critical to the understanding of many disease processes, a feature that renders vague the distinction of a particular pathology as simply neurological, immunological, or endocrinological. For instance, Alzheimer's disease is characterized by the presence of beta-amyloid protein deposits, neurofibrillary tangles, and cholinergic dysfunction throughout the hippocampal region. It has been postulated that the structural and metabolic damage found in Alzheimer's disease is secondary to sustained elevation of IL-1beta, a feature that is also found in type 1 diabetes mellitus (Holden and Mooney, 1995). IL-1beta and IL-6, but not IL-2, contents are significantly elevated in the cerebrospinal fluid (CSF), but not plasma, of de novo Parkinson's disease and Alzheimer's disease patients as compared to controls. Because IL-1beta and IL-6 play a key role in the interaction between the nervous and immune system, e.g., in the so-called acute phase response, these observations support the involvement of immunological events in the complex process of neurodegeneration in Alzheimer's and Parkinson's diseases (Blum-Degen et al., 1995).

IL-1beta has anorectic, hyperthermic, and analgesic or hyperalgesic (depending on the studies) effects in the rat. IL-1beta has anorectic affects in three diencephalic sites (the perifornical area, an area above the optic chiasma, and an area internal to the mamillothalamic tract). IL-1beta has hyperthermic effects in seven sites (the media and lateral preoptic area, the hypothalamic periventricular substance, the dorso-medial and arcuate nuclei of the hypothalamus, and the centromedial and gelatinosus nuclei of the thalamus). IL-1beta has analgesic effects in the centromedial and gelatinosus nuclei of the thalamus. IL-1beta also increases food intake and decreases pain sensation thresholds in the paraventricular nucleus of the hypothalamus (Sellami and de Beaurepaire, 1995). Under physiological conditions, rat hippocampal neurons in culture concomitantly release IL-1beta and IFN-gamma; under anoxic conditions, the increase in IL-1beta release is paralleled by a decrease in IFN-gamma levels. The latter anoxic injury-associated cytokine expression pattern is reverted to the physiological pattern by the addition of 2-amino-5-phosphonopentanoate, an N-methyl-D-aspartate receptor antagonist (Pellegrini et al., 1996), an observation which suggests that IFN-gamma may have a physiological regulating role in the IL-1 neurotoxic action and homeostasis recovery following an insult.

Growth-factor induction is also a major component of the response to central nervous system (CNS) trauma. The insulin-like growth factors (IGFs) and IGF-binding proteins (IGFBPs) are among the molecules induced by injury that have demonstrated neuroprotective actions. IGFBP2 is uniquely upregulated among the IGFBPs in the central nervous system (CNS) and is induced by cytokines, such as ciliary neurotrophic factor (CNTF) and IL-1beta, that signal CNS injury (Wood et al., 1995). The nerve growth factor that induces phenotypic changes in PC12 pheochromocytoma cells also induces the expression of the proinflammatory cytokine IL-1alpha in these cells (Alheim et al., 1996). IL-1Ra increases survival during rat heatstroke by reducing hypothalamic serotonin release (Chiu et al., 1995). Analysis of IL-1beta and IL-1 receptor expression in mice shows an age-related reciprocal modulation in the hippocampus (Takao et al., 1996).

NEUROENDOCRINOLOGY OF CHRONIC FATIGUE SYNDROME

The study of CFS has also benefited from multidisciplinary assessments in which immune, endocrine, and neurological variables have been studied. The main system dysfunction is not clear, but a unified picture is slowly emerging from the studies performed. For example, Kavelaars et al. (2000) point out that CFS is accompanied by a relative resistance of the immune system to regulation by the neuroendocrine system, as evidenced by a reduction in the sensitivity of the immune system to the glucocorticoid agonist dexamethasone and the beta2-adrenergic agonist terbutaline in fifteen adolescent girls with CFS as compared to fourteen age- and sex-matched controls. Kavelaars et al. (2000) suggest that CFS should be viewed as a disease of deficient neuroendocrine-immune communication.

A rationale for the study of neuroendocrine correlates of CFS stems from the observation that fatigue states share many of the somatic symptom characteristics seen in recognized endocrine disorders (Anisman et al., 1996; Baschetti, 1996, 1997; Demitrack, 1997, 1998; Jones et al., 1998; Korszun et al., 1998; Poteliakhoff, 1998; Sterzl and Zamrazil, 1996). Moreover, patients with CFS or fibromyalgia with chronic facial pain show a high comorbidity with other stress-associated syndromes (e.g., irritable bowel syndrome, premenstrual syndrome, and interstitial cystitis) and autoimmune conditions associated with endocrinological dysfunction. Therefore, the clinical overlap between these conditions may reflect a shared underlying pathophysiologic basis involving dysregulation of the hypothalamic-pituitary-adrenal (HPA) stress hormone axis in predisposed individuals (Anisman et al., 1996; Baschetti, 1996, 1997, 1999a,b,c,d; Demitrack, 1997, 1998; Heim et al., 2000; Jeffcoate, 1999; Jones et al., 1998; Korszun et al., 1998; Poteliakhoff, 1998; Pruessner et al., 1999; Scott and Dinan, 1999; Scott, Medbak, et al., 1999; Scott, Salahuddin, et al., 1999; Scott, Reznek, et al., 1999; Sterzl and Zamrazil, 1996).

Several reports have provided replicated evidence of disruptions in the integrity of the HPA axis in CFS patients. It is notable that the pattern of alteration in the stress response apparatus is not reminiscent of the well-understood hypercortisolism of melancholic depression but rather suggests a sustained inactivation of CNS components of this system. In this respect, one report documented a significantly lower urinary free cortisol (UFC) excretion in CFS patients and a significantly higher UFC excretion in patients with depression as compared to controls (Scott and Dinan, 1998). A subgroup of CFS patients with comorbid depressive illness retained the pattern of UFC excretion of those with CFS alone, an observation that points to a different pathophysiological basis for depressive symptoms in CFS. Another study further confirmed cortisol hyposecretion in saliva as well as plasma of CFS patients, compared to patients with depression and controls (Strickland et al., 1998). A study by Scott, Salahuddin, et al. (1999) found that dehydro-epiandrosterone (DHEA) and DHEA-sulphate (DHEA-S) levels were significantly lower in CFS patients compared to controls; in contrast, DHEA-S levels, but not DHEA, were lower in depressives; cortisol and 17-alpha-hydroxyprogesterone did not differ between the three groups. De Becker et al. (1999) found normal basal DHEA levels but a blunted DHEA response curve to intravenous ACTH injection.

Study of the detailed, pulsatile characteristics of the HPA axis in CFS patients revealed a reduction of HPA axis activity due, in part, to impaired CNS drive (Demitrack and Crofford, 1998). A diminished output of neurotrophic adrenocorticotropic hormone (ACTH) in response to administration of 100 μg of ovine corticotropin-releasing hormone (CRH), causing a reduced adrenocortical secretory reserve that is inadequately compensated for by adrenoceptor upregulation, is suggested to explain the reduced cortisol production in CFS patients (Scott et al., 1998a). Using the 1 μg ACTH test, another study provided further evidence for a subtle pituitary-adrenal insufficiency (lower delta cortisol value) in CFS patients compared to controls (Scott et al., 1998b). Measurement of ACTH and cortisol responses following the administration of the opiate antagonist naloxone revealed that naloxone-mediated activation of the HPA axis is attenuated in CFS, an observation that renders excessive opioid inhibition of the HPA axis an unlikely explanation for its dysregulation in this disorder (Scott, Burnett, et al., 1998). Scott, Reznek, et al. (1999) reported a reduction of over 50 percent in the size of both adrenal glands in eight CFS subjects with a subnormal ACTH response, an observation that is indicative of significant adrenal atrophy in this group of CFS patients.

Several studies disagree with the findings previously described. One study found a significantly decreased diurnal change in cortisol levels, and nonsignificant lower levels of morning cortisol and higher levels of ACTH and evening cortisol among CFS patients as compared to controls (MacHale et al., 1998). Although a relationship between adrenocortical function and disability in CFS (general health and physical functioning, functional improvement over the last year, and current social functioning) was found, no causal connection was apparent. Another study failed to document a reduction in the basal activity of the HPA axis in measurements of salivary and urinary cortisol over a twenty-four-hour period (Young et al., 1998). One study found slightly but significantly higher mean levels of salivary cortisol (hourly sampling over a sixteen-hour period) in CFS patients as compared to controls (Wood et al., 1998). Hudson and Cleare (1999) have pointed out that the inconsistencies in studies assessing the HPA axis may be secondary to heterogeneity in the presence of sleep disturbances, inactivity, altered circadian rhythmicity, illness chronicity, concomitant medication, and comorbid psychiatric disturbance.

Other work also implicates alterations in central serotonergic tone in the overall pathophysiology of HPA axis dysregulation (Sharpe et al., 1997). One study found that release of ACTH (but not cortisol) in response to ipsapirone (20 mg orally) was significantly blunted in patients with CFS, and concluded that serotonergic activation of the HPA axis is defective in CFS (Dinan et al., 1997). Scott, Medbak, et al. (1999) reported that desmopressin (DDAVP), which augments CRH-mediated pituitary-adrenal responsivity in healthy subjects, was capable of normalizing the pituitary-adrenal response to CRH in CFS patients. The latter observation suggests that there may be increased vasopressinergic responsivity of the anterior pituitary in CFS and/or that DDAVP may be exerting an effect at an adrenal level (Scott, Medbak, et al., 1999).

In terms of the growth hormone/insulin-like growth factor (IGF)-1(somatomedin C) axis, one study found that, in contrast to patients with fibromyalgia, in whom levels of somatomedin C have been found to be reduced, levels in patients with CFS were found to be elevated. Thus, despite the clinical similarities between these two conditions, they may be associated with different abnormalities of sleep and/or the somatotropic neuroendocrine axis (Bennett, Mayes, et al., 1997; Berwaerts et al., 1998; Buchwald, Umali, et al., 1996). Another study found attenuated basal levels of IGF-I and IGF-II in CFS patients and a reduced GH response to hypoglycemia (Allain et al., 1997). Insulin levels were higher and IGF-binding protein-1 (IGFBP1) levels were lower in CFS patients compared with controls. Unlike the latter reports, no significant differences were observed among any of three patient groups (CFS, fibromyalgia, and patients with both), and controls in the mean concentration of either IGF-I or IGFBP3 in another study (Vara-Thorbeck et al., 1996). Cleare et al. (2000) also failed to find evidence for abnormalities in the IGF-1/GH hormone axis.

The implications of observations of neuroendocrine dysfunction are an area of intense research, and interesting correlations and therapeutic interventions are being formulated. For instance, one group found that the previously described relationships in healthy women between basal circulating neutrophil numbers and plasma progesterone concentrations and between exercise-induced neutrophilia and urinary cortisol and plasma creatine kinase concentrations were not observed in CFS women, observations that suggest normal endocrine influences on the circulating neutrophil pool may be disrupted in CFS patients (Cannon et al., 1998). Moreover, the differential sensitivity of cytokine expression by CD4 T-cell subsets in CFS patients to glucocorticoids might explain an altered immunologic function in CFS patients (Visser et al., 1998). However, LaManca et al. (1999) found that the immunological response to an exhaustive treadmill exercise test in twenty female chronic fatigue syndrome patients did not differ with that of fourteen matched sedentary controls.

Because changes in both endocrine and immune status variables are observed in CFS, it is noteworthy that during acute febrile illness immune-derived cytokines initiate an acute phase response, which is characterized by fever, inactivity, fatigue, anorexia, and catabolism. Profound neuroendocrine and metabolic changes also take place: acute phase proteins are produced in the liver, bone marrow function and the metabolic activity of leukocytes are greatly increased, and specific immune reactivity is suppressed. Defects in regulatory processes, which are fundamental to immune disorders and inflammatory diseases, may lie in the immune system, the neuroendocrine system, or both. Baschetti (1999a) has proposed that cortisol deficiency may account for elevated apoptotic cell population proportions in CFS patients. Defects in the HPA axis have been observed in autoimmune and rheumatic diseases and chronic inflammatory disease. Prolactin levels are often elevated in patients with systemic lupus erythematosus and other autoimmune diseases, whereas the bioactivity of prolactin is decreased in patients with rheumatoid arthritis. Levels of sex hormones and thyroid hormone are decreased during severe inflammatory disease. Defective neural regulation of inflammation likely plays a pathogenic role in allergy and asthma, in the symmetrical form of rheumatoid arthritis and in gastrointestinal inflammatory disease.

Based on the different observations previously described, Pall (2000) has proposed another unifying hypothesis of CFS in which either viral or bacterial infection induces one or more cytokines, IL-1beta, IL-6, TNF-alpha, and IFN-gamma. The latter cytokines induce nitric oxide synthase (iNOS), leading to increased nitric oxide levels. Nitric oxide, in turn, reacts with superoxide radical to generate the potent oxidant peroxynitrite. Pall (2000) proposed multiple amplification and positive feedback mechanisms by which once peroxynitrite levels are elevated, they tend to be sustained at a high level. The latter proposed mechanism may lower the HPA axis activity and be maintained by consequent lowered glucocorticoid levels.

The studies of the interactions between the immune, endocrine, and nervous systems are fertile ground for applications not only to the understanding and therapy of CFS but also to those of other diseases. A better understanding of neuroimmunoregulation holds the promise of new approaches to the treatment of immune and inflammatory diseases with the use of hormones, neurotransmitters, neuropeptides, and drugs that modulate these regulators (Anisman et al., 1996). For instance, an article proposes a possible common pathophysiology and treatment with replacement of depleted brain dopamine for postpolio fatigue and CFS based on the clinically significant deficits on neuropsychologic tests of attention, histopathologic and neuroradiologic evidence of brain lesions, impaired activation of the HPA axis, increased prolactin secretion, and electroencephalogram slow-wave activity seen in both conditions (Bruno et al., 1998). Some therapeutic attempts have not yielded clear-cut results, but have provided further insight into the neuroendocrinology of CFS. For instance, acute administration of the serotonin receptor agonist buspirone (0.5 mg/kg orally) in eleven male patients with CFS and a group of matched healthy controls showed that CFS patients had significantly higher plasma prolactin concentrations and experienced more nausea in response to buspirone than did controls (Sharpe et al., 1996). However, the growth hormone response to buspirone did not distinguish CFS patients from controls. The latter data question whether the enhancement of buspirone-induced prolactin release in CFS is a consequence of increased sensitivity of postsynaptic serotonin receptors but open the possibility that it could reflect changes in dopamine function

(Sharpe et al., 1996). Although hydrocortisone treatment (13 mg/m^2 of body surface area every morning and 3 mg/m^2 every afternoon for twelve weeks) in a randomized, placebo-controlled, double-blind therapeutic trial was associated with some improvement in symptoms of CFS (as assessed by Wellness scale), the degree of adrenal suppression (twelve out of thirty patients) precludes its practical use for CFS (McKenzie et al., 1998). Low-dose hydrocortisone treatment in chronic fatigue syndrome has been assessed and recommended by some authors (Baschetti, 1999,b,c; Cleare et al., 1999; Friedman et al., 1999; Teitelbaum et al., 1999).

Chapter 3

The Soldiers of the Immune Army: Immune Cell Phenotypic Distributions

Although the cause of CFS remains to be elucidated and the previous chapters illustrated many of the neuroendocrinological changes in CFS, many studies have also provided evidence for abnormalities in immunological markers among individuals diagnosed with CFS. A clear picture has not been achieved because of the noticeable variability in the nature and magnitude of the findings reported by different groups (Patarca et al., 1992; Sobel et al., 1988). Moreover, little support has been garnered for an association between the latter abnormalities and the diverse physical and health status changes in the CFS population. For instance, Buchwald and co-workers (1997) concluded that although a subset of CFS patients with immune system activation can be identified, serum markers of inflammation and immune activation are of limited diagnostic usefulness in the evaluation of patients with CFS and chronic fatigue because changes in their values may reflect an intercurrent, transient, common condition, such as an upper-respiratory infection, or may be the result of an ongoing illness-associated process. On the other hand, Patarca and colleagues (Patarca, Klimas, Sandler, et al., 1995) have found that CFS patients can be categorized based on immunological findings. It is also worth noting that although the degree of overlap between distributions of soluble immune mediators in CFS and controls has fueled criticism on the validity or clinical significance of immune abnormalities in CFS, the latter degree of overlap is not unique to CFS and is also present, for instance, in sepsis syndrome and HIV-1-associated disease, clinical entities in which studies of immune abnormalities are providing insight into pathophysiology (Goldie et al., 1995).

Analysis of the complex interactions underlying immune responses was greatly facilitated by the development of monoclonal antibodies to various surface proteins on lymphoid cells, which defined functionally distinct subsets (Cantor and Boyse, 1977; Reinherz and Schlossman, 1981; Romain and Schlossman, 1984). Such analysis has also demonstrated that each type of lymphoid cell is genetically programmed to carry out defined immunological functions that are predictable on the basis of surface phenotype (Romain and Schlossman, 1984).

Surface-marker phenotyping of peripheral blood lymphoid cells has also allowed insight into the cellular basis of immune dysfunction associated with pathologies of many organ systems with diverse causes, including viral, autoimmune, and genetic, among others (see, for example, Calabrese et al, 1987; Fletcher et al., 1989; Griffin, 1991; Klimas, Morgan, et al., 1992; Klimas, Patarca, et al., 1992; McAllister et al., 1989; Raziuddin and Elawad, 1990; Villemain et al., 1989). Several reports also documented alterations in the distribution of various lymphoid cell subsets among CFS patients. Certain discrepancies in the findings from different study groups can be attributed to group nonequivalences on diverse parameters such as demographic variables (gender, age, socioeconomic status), medical status variables predating onset of disease, medication use, concomitant substance abuse, nutritional status, and the effects of time of sample collection (diurnal or seasonal variations) (Fletcher et al., 1989; Herberman, 1991; Lahita, 1982; Malone et al., 1990; Martin et al., 1988; Patarca, Sandler, et al., 1995; Roberts et al., 1998; Schulte, 1991; Whiteside, 1994). Methodological flaws are also to blame because some studies used frozen cells in their assessments, and cryopreservation is known to affect the expression of many surface markers and cytokines.

T LYMPHOCYTES

CD4+ T cells (helper-inducer cells) are the principal source of "help" for antibody production by B cells in response to T-cell-dependent antigenic stimulation, as well as inducers of cytotoxic and suppressor T-cell function (CD8+ cells; Reinherz and Schlossman, 1981). Discrepant results have been reported in reference to CD4+ and CD8+ cell counts in CFS patients. Straus and colleagues (1985) reported a statistically higher percentage of CD4+ lymphocytes with normal numbers of CD8+ cells and CD4/CD8 ratio; Jones (1991), Jones and Straus (1987), Jones and colleagues (1985),

Borysiewicz et al. (1986), Gupta and Vayuvegula (1991), Landay et al. (1991), Lloyd et al. (1992), and Tirelli et al. (1994) found normal percentages of CD4+ and CD8+ cells as well as a normal CD4/CD8 ratio; Lloyd and co-authors (1989) found decreased numbers of both CD4+ and CD8+ cells; Buchwald and Komaroff (1991) found reduced numbers of CD8+ cells and higher-than-normal CD4/CD8 ratios; and Klimas and colleagues (1990) found that most CFS subjects studied had a normal number of CD4+ cells and an elevated number of CD8+ cells which resulted in a decrease in the CD4/CD8 ratio (Klimas et al., 1990). Decreased CD4/CD8 ratios in 2 to 100 percent of patients have been demonstrated by other investigators (Aoki et al., 1987; DuBois, 1986; Jones et al., 1985; Jones and Straus, 1987; Jones, 1991; Linde et al., 1988).

These conflicting results may be associated with the fluctuation in clinical manifestations of these patients or with other factors mentioned previously. In fact, several researchers have detected fluctuations in several immunological parameters and in the severity of symptoms in longitudinal follow-up investigations of patients with CFS. Moreover, Mawle and co-workers (1997) found that although only marginal differences in cytokine responses and in cell surface markers were apparent in the total CFS population they studied, when the patients were subgrouped by type of disease onset (gradual or sudden) or by how well they were feeling on the day of testing, more pronounced differences were seen. It is also worth noting that although Peakman and co-workers (1997) did not find significant differences in the percentage levels of total CD3+, CD4+, CD8+, and activated, naive, and memory T-cell subsets between CFS subjects and controls, they cryopreserved the cells before flow cytometric analysis, and cryopreservation can differentially affect the representation of T-cell subsets (Patarca, Goodkin, et al., 1995).

A study by Sandman and colleagues (1992) found that elevated CD4+ and CD8+ cell counts in CFS patients were related to decreases in priming of memory and speed of memory scanning, and increases in errors on a memory fragility test. However, the latter study did not control for depression severity, and it is not clear whether the finding is related to comorbid depression or to CFS itself.

Klimas and co-workers (1990) found a decreased proportion of CD4+CD45RA+ cells, which are associated with suppressor/cytotoxic cell induction (Morimoto et al., 1985), but Natelson and co-workers (1998) found no significant change in the proportions of CD4+CD45RA+ and CD4+CD45RO+ cells in CFS patients. Franco and colleagues (1987) also described a decrease in the number of CD4+CD45RA+ lymphocytes in two patients with severe, chronic, active Epstein-Barr virus (EBV) infection; one of the two patients showed a persistent diminished number of cells despite clinical improvement with IL-2 treatment. Several publications have associated alterations in the latter subset with a number of clinical entities, particularly autoimmune diseases (Alpert et al., 1987; Emery et al., 1987; Klimas, Morgan, et al., 1992; Morimoto et al., 1985; Sato et al., 1987; Sobel et al., 1988). In a study of lymph node and peripheral blood lymphocytes, Fletcher et al. (2000) also reported decreased proportion of naive T cells in both lymph node and peripheral blood. They also found that in CFS patients, as in normal controls, approximately 80 percent of lymph node lymphocytes are CD3+, of which over 65 percent are CD4+ (Black et al., 1980; Bryan et al., 1993; Kelly-Williams et al., 1989; Lindelman et al., 1983; Tedla et al., 1999). Moreover, the proportion of CD8+ lymph node lymphocytes found in CFS patients is in the midrange of values reported for control individuals (Black et al., 1980; Bryan et al., 1993; Kelly-Williams et al., 1989; Lindelman et al., 1983; Tedla et al., 1999). The variance of CD8+ cell proportions among the different studies may be related to the specific location of the nodes studied, the status of nodal reactivity at the time of harvest, the technique used to make the lymphocyte suspensions, as well as the methods of staining and analysis (Tedla et al., 1999).

Increased numbers of T cells expressing the activation marker CD26, probably as a result of CD8+ activation, have also been reported in CFS patients (Klimas et al., 1990). In this respect, an increased proportion of CD8+ cells expressing the activation marker human leukocyte antigen (HLA)-DR (Barker et al., 1994; Hassan et al., 1998; Klimas et al., 1990; Landay et al., 1991) have been reported in CFS patients, whereas normal proportions of CD4+ T cells coexpressing the HLA-DR marker or the IL-2 receptor (CD25) were found in one study (Landay et al., 1991), normal proportions of CD8+ CD38+, CD8+CD11b-, CD8+HLA-DR+, and CD8+CD28+ were found in another study (Natelson et al., 1998), and normal proportions of CD8+HLA-DR+ and CD8+CD38+ were found by Swanink and co-workers (Swanink et al., 1996). In contrast to the latter findings, Hassan and colleagues (1998) found significantly decreased expression of CD28 on CD8 cells and Barker and colleagues (1994), Landay and colleagues (1991), and Swanink et al. (1996) found significantly decreased expression of CD11b on CD8 cells. Higher expression of CD38 on CD8 cells was found by Barker et al. (1994), Landay et al. (1991), and Peakman et al. (1997).

It is worth noting that relatively higher proportions of HLA-DR+ T cells have been reported in a number of autoimmune disorders (Alviggi et al., 1984; Canonica et al., 1982; Jackson et al., 1984; Koide, 1985; Rabinowe et al., 1984), and that Hassan and co-workers (1998) found that CFS patients with increased HLA-DR expression had significantly lower Short Form-36 health questionnaire (SF-36) total scores, worse body pains, and poorer general health perception and physical functioning scores. The increased expression of class II antigens and the reduced expression of the costimulatory receptor CD28, which is a marker of terminally differentiated cells, lend further support to the concept of immunoactivation of T lymphocytes in CFS and may be consistent with the notion of a viral etiopathogenesis in the illness.

A study of the association between CFS physical symptoms, illness burden, and lymphocyte activation markers in twenty-seven newly recruited CFS patients (Helder et al., 1998) revealed that elevations in T-helper/inducer cells were associated with a greater frequency and severity of tender lymph nodes, greater severity of memory and concentration difficulties, and headaches. Greater numbers of activated T cells (CD2+CD3+CD26+) were associated with a greater frequency of tender lymph nodes and cognitive difficulties, and more activated cytotoxic/suppressor cells (CD8+CD38+HLA-DR+) were associated with greater severity of tender lymph nodes, fatigue, and sleep problems. Conversely, lower percentages of regulatory cells such as CD3+CD8+ were associated with a greater number of cognitive difficulties, greater Sickness Impact Profile (SIP) Total, SIP Physical Impairment, and an increased frequency and severity of memory problems, increased frequency of headaches, and increased severity of fatigue. Thus, among CFS patients the degree of cellular immune activation is associated with the severity of CFS-related physical symptoms, cognitive complaints, and perceived illness burden.

B LYMPHOCYTES

Gupta and Vayuvegula (1991), Klimas et al. (1990), Landay et al. (1991), Lloyd et al. (1992), and Barker et al. (1994) found normal levels of CD20+ resting B cells, whereas other teams reported both increased and decreased levels (Borysiewicz et al., 1986; Buchwald and Komaroff, 1991; Linde et al., 1988; Tirelli et al., 1994). The proportion of CD5-bearing B cells was found to be increased in two studies (Klimas et al., 1990; Tirelli et al., 1994), and decreased in one study (Landay et al., 1991). B cells bearing the cell marker CD5 have been associated with autoimmunity (Casali and Notkins, 1989).

NATURAL KILLER CELLS

Klimas et al. (1990), Morrison et al. (1991), Peakman et al. (1997), and Tirelli et al. (1994) found increased numbers of NK cells, whereas Barker et al. (1994), Landay et al. (1991), Lloyd et al. (1992), and Natelson et al. (1998) found normal numbers and Masuda et al. (1994) and Gupta et al. (1991) found decreased numbers of NK cells. Despite the discrepancy in total numbers of NK cells measured by different groups, Caligiuri et al. (1987) and Morrison et al. (1991) found an increased proportion of CD56+CD3+ T cells, which may account for the decreased natural killer (NK) cell cytotoxic activity seen in several studies of CFS patients. Morrison and co-workers (1991) also found a decreased percentage of CD56+Fcgamma receptor+ NK cells, which suggests a reduced capacity for antibody-dependent cellular toxicity.

NEUTROPHILS

Previously described relationships in healthy women between basal circulating neutrophil numbers and plasma progesterone concentrations and between exercise-induced neutrophilia and urinary cortisol and plasma creatine kinase concentrations, were not observed in CFS women. Observations that suggest normal endocrine influences on the circulating neutrophil pool may be disrupted in CFS patients (Cannon et al., 1998).

Chapter 4

Immune Cell Function

T AND B LYMPHOCYTES

Depressed responses to phytohemagglutinin (PHA) and pokeweed mitogen (PWM), an indication of dysfunction in cellular immunity, were found in the CFS patients studied by most teams (Aoki et al., 1987; Behan et al., 1985; Borysiewicz et al., 1986; Hassan et al., 1998; Jones et al., 1985; Jones and Straus, 1987; Jones, 1991; Klimas et al., 1990; Lloyd et al., 1989, 1992; Straus et al., 1985; Tobi et al., 1982). Mawle and co-workers (1997) found no change. Gupta and Vayuvegula (1991) found that the lymphocyte DNA synthesis in response to PHA, PWM, and concanavalin A was normal in CFS patients, but the response to soluble antigens (mumps, *E. coli*) was significantly reduced. Roberts and colleagues (1998) found that the degree of PWM-induced lymphoproliferative response is associated with Rh status among healthy controls but not among CFS patients, and recommended to control future studies for Rh status. In terms of the functional implications of decreased lymphoproliferative activities in CFS, Hassan and co-workers (1998) reported that PHA proliferative responses were lower in patients with poor emotional and mental health scores, and the anti-CD3/anti-CD28 response was low in those with low general health perception scores. T-cell dysfunction in CFS patients has been suggested to result from decreased surface expression of CD3, an important component of the T-cell receptor complex (Subira et al., 1989), and Barker and co-workers (1994) found no significant increase in the mean proliferation of peripheral blood cells when stimulated with the anti-CD3 antibody.

In terms of the impaired lymphocyte responses seen in CFS patients, Bounous and Molson (1999) pointed out that, as an antioxidant, glutathione (GSH) is essential for allowing the lymphocyte to express its full potential without being hampered by oxiradical accumulation. Hence, protracted challenge of the immunocytes may lead to cellular GSH depletion. Bounous and Molson (1999) hypothesized that because GSH is also essential to aerobic muscular contraction, an undesirable competition for GSH precursors between the immune and muscular systems may develop. It is conceivable that the priority of the immune system for the survival of the host has drawn to this vital area the ever-diminishing GSH precursors, thus depriving the skeletal muscle of adequate GSH precursors to sustain a normal aerobic metabolism resulting in fatigue and eventually myalgia (Bounous and Molson, 1999).

In terms of B-cell function, spontaneous and mitogen-induced immunoglobulin synthesis is also affected. Despite these deficits in B-cell function, stimulation with allergens provides differential lymphocyte responsiveness. Greater in vitro lymphocyte responses to specific allergens, greater baseline levels of lymphocyte incorporation of tritiated thymidine, and an increased number of immunoglobulin E-bearing B and T lymphocytes have been reported (Olson, Kanaan, Gersuk, et al., 1986; Olson, Kanaan, Kelley, et al., 1986). Elevation in levels of certain cytokines, such as IL-4, IL-5, and IL-6 may underlie the latter effects. In a sample of sixty-five CFS patients, Lutgendorf, Antoni, et al. (1995) and Lutgendorf, Klimas, et al. (1995) observed that decreased lymphoproliferative responses to PHA and PWM were associated with increased cognitive difficulties and greater SIP physical illness burden.

Another area of research in CFS is that of apoptosis, the process of programmed cell death, which is regulated by several genes including Bax and Bcl-2. The Bcl-2 protein forms a heterodimer with Bax that inhibits apoptosis, whereas the Bax-Bax homodimer promotes it. A report by Hassan and co-workers (1998) on surface and intracellular immunologic and apoptotic markers and functional lymphocyte assays after stimulation with anti-CD3/anti-CD28 antibodies or PHA in forty-four CFS patients revealed increased expression of the apoptosis repressor ratio of Bcl-2/Bax in both CD4 and CD8. However, recent evidence indicates that induction of apoptosis might be mediated in a dysregulated immune system, such as that present in CFS, by the up-regulation of growth inhibitory cytokines. In this respect, Vojdani and colleagues (1997) found an increased apoptotic cell population in CFS individuals as compared to healthy controls. The increased apoptotic subpopulation in CFS individuals was accompanied by an abnormal cell arrest in the S phase and the G2/M boundary of the cell cycle as compared to the control group. In addition, CFS individuals exhibited enhanced mRNA and protein levels of the IFN-induced protein kinase RNA (PKR) product as compared to healthy controls. In 50 percent of the CFS samples treated with 2-aminopurine (a potent inhibitor of PKR) the apoptotic population was reduced by more than 50 percent. PKR-mediated apoptosis may thus contribute to the pathogenesis and the fatigue symptomatology associated with CFS. See and colleagues (1998) found that the addition of a glyconutrient compound (dietary supplement that supplies the eight crucial monosaccharides required for synthesis of glycoproteins) to peripheral blood cells of CFS patients in vitro significantly decreased the percentage of apoptotic cells (all three parameters were deficient at baseline).

In contrast to the studies previously described, Swanink and coworkers (1996) found no obvious difference in apoptosis in leukocyte cultures from CFS patients.

NATURAL KILLER CELLS

Several studies revealed impaired NK cell function in CFS patients as assessed by cytotoxic activity against K562 cells (Barker et al., 1994; Caligiuri et al., 1987; DuBois, 1986; Kibler et al., 1985; Klimas et al., 1990; Ojo-Amaise et al., 1994; See et al., 1997; Straus et al., 1985; Whiteside and Friberg, 1998) and a decreased number of CD56+CD3– lymphocytes (Caligiuri et al., 1987; Morrison et al., 1991). A study by Levine and co-workers (1998) on NK cell activity in a family with members who had developed CFS as adults, as compared to those who had not, documented low NK cell activity in six out of eight cases and in four out of twelve unaffected family members. Two of the offspring of the CFS cases had pediatric malignancies. Based on these observations, the authors suggested that the low NK cell activity in this family may be a result of a genetically determined immunologic abnormality predisposing to CFS and cancer. Gold and colleagues (1990) were the only group to find elevated NK cell activity among the CFS patients they studied, whereas Mawle and colleagues (1997) found no change in NK cell function.

The changes in NK cell cytotoxic activity found by most groups could be related to several findings: (1) CD56+CD3– cells are the lymphoid subset with highest NK cell activity, and a decrease in their representation is expected to lower the value for the NK cell activity per effector cells; (2) the reduction in CD4+CD45+ T cells described previously may also result in decreased induction of suppressor/ cytotoxic T cells; and (3) reduced NK cell activity may be associated with deficiencies in the production of IL-2 and interferon (IFN)-gamma by T cells or in the ability of NK cells to respond to these lymphokines. In the terms of the latter possibility, Buchwald and Komaroff (1991) found that stimulation with IL-2 failed to result in improvement of cytolytic activity in many patients with CFS.

Poor NK cell function may also be related to the finding of an impaired ability of lymphocytes from CFS patients to produce IFN-gamma in response to mitogenic stimuli (Kibler et al., 1985; Klimas et al., 1990). Although one study reported elevated IFN-gamma production (Altman et al., 1988) and another demonstrated normal production (Morte et al., 1988), the inability of lymphocytes from CFS patients to produce IFN-gamma found by Klimas et al. (1990), Kibler et al. (1985), and Visser et al. (1998) might represent a cellular exhaustion as a consequence of persistent viral stimulus. The latter postulate is supported by Morag et al. (1982) and Straus et al.'s (1985) finding of elevated levels of leukocyte 2'5'-oligoadenylate synthetase, an IFN-inducible enzyme, in lymphocytes of CFS patients. Furthermore, the lack of IFN-gamma production in CFS patients may be responsible for the impaired activation of immunoregulatory circuits, which in turn facilitates the reactivation and progression of viral infections. In this respect, Lusso and associates (1987) described the prevention of intercellular spread of EBV mediated by the IFN released as a consequence of cellular response, and Borysiewicz and co-workers (1986) described normal NK cell activity but reduced EBV-specific cytotoxic T-cell activity in their CFS patients. Reactivation/replication of a latent virus (such as Epstein-Barr virus) secondary to decreased NK cell activity has also been proposed to modulate the immune system to induce CFS (Glaser and Kiecolt-Glaser, 1998).

More recent research has provided alternative explanations for the decreased NK cell activity observed in CFS. A study by Ogawa and co-workers (1998) revealed a possible dysfunction in the nitric oxide (NO)-mediated NK cell activation in CFS patients based on the observations that twenty-four-hour treatment of NK cells with L-Arginine (L-Arg), one of the essential amino acids, enhanced NK cell activity in controls, but not in CFS patients. Although the expression of inducible NO synthase (iNOS) (the enzyme involved in the synthesis of NO from L-Arg) transcripts in peripheral blood mononuclear cells was not significantly different between healthy control subjects and CFS patients, and incubation with S-nitroso-N-acetylpenicillamine, an NO donor, stimulated NK cell activity in healthy control subjects but not in CFS patients. See and co-workers (1998) reported that addition in vitro of a glyconutrient compound (dietary supplement that supplies the eight crucial monosaccharides required for synthesis of glycoproteins) to peripheral blood cells from CFS patients significantly enhanced natural killer cell activity, increased the expression of the glycoproteins CD5, CD8, and CD11a, and decreased the percentage of apoptotic cells, parameters that were all deficient at baseline. The latter observation would be consistent with a defect in glycoprotein synthesis.

See and Tilles (1996) treated thirty CFS patients IFN-alpha 2a or placebo in a double-blind crossover study. Outcome was evaluated by NK cell function, lymphocyte proliferation to mitogens and soluble antigens, CD4/CD8 counts, and a ten-item Quality of Life (QOL) survey. Although mean NK function increased after twelve weeks of IFN therapy, there was no significant change in the other immunologic parameters or QOL scores. When the twenty-six patients who completed the study were stratified according to their baseline NK cell function and lymphocyte proliferation, four groups were identified: three patients had normal NK cell function and lymphocyte proliferation when compared to normal, healthy controls; nine had isolated deficiency in lymphocyte proliferation; seven had diminished NK function only; and seven had abnormalities for both parameters. QOL scores were not significantly different for the four groups at baseline. After twelve weeks of interferon therapy, QOL score significantly improved in each of the seven patients with isolated NK cell dysfunction compared to baseline. In these patients the mean NK cell function increased. Significant improvement was not recorded for QOL in the other three groups. Thus, therapy with IFN-alpha has a significant effect on the QOL of that subgroup of patients with CFS manifesting an isolated decrease in NK cell function.

Pursuing the hypothesis that the low-grade fever and fatigue in low NK syndrome (LNKS)—a condition resembling CFS in many but not all ways (Aoki et al., 1985, 1987)—might be abrogated by interventions that normalize NK functioning, one group has tested the effects of immunopotentiators with patients diagnosed with LNKS. They found in single-blind trials (contents of medication were not revealed to patients) that although the administration of antipyretics, nonsteroidal anti-inflammatory drugs or antibiotics had no detectable effects on fever, lentinan (a glucon extracted from Japanese mushrooms), improved clinical symptoms and increased natural killer cell cytotoxicity (NKCC) and antibody-dependent cellular cytotoxicity (ADCC) in patients with LNKS (Miyakoshi et al., 1984). Although preliminary, this is one of the only studies to document parallel improvement in CFS-like clinical symptoms and NKCC following an experimental manipulation. However, this study did not focus specifically on CDC-diagnosed CFS patients.

MONOCYTES

Prieto and co-authors (Prieto et al., 1989) found significant monocyte dysfunction in patients with CFS, such as reduced display of vimentin, phagocytosis index, and surface expression of HLA-DR. These deficits responded to naloxone treatment, which suggests that increased interaction of endogenous opioids with monocyte receptors might account for the monocyte dysfunction. Gupta and co-workers (1997) found that monocytes from CFS patients display an increased density of ICAM-1 and LFA-1, but showed decreased enhancing response to recombinant IFN-gamma in vitro. In contrast to the latter studies, Barker and co-workers (1994) did not find abnormalities in superoxide anion production and phagocytosis in CFS patients. Moreover, lack of a consistent elevation of neopterin, a macrophage activation marker (see Eosinophils), suggests that monocytes do not appear to account for the imbalances in IL-1.

EOSINOPHILS

Conti and colleagues (1996) provided evidence for eosinophil activation in CFS by demonstrating elevated serum levels of eosinophil cationic protein (ECP). In the CFS population they studied, the prevalence of reaction allergen-specific testing (RAST) positivity to one or more allergens was 77 percent, and no control showed positive RAST. Twelve of the fourteen CFS patients with increased ECP serum levels were RAST positive. However, CFS RAST-positive patients had no significantly higher ECP serum levels than CFS RAST-negative patients. It remains to be determined whether eosinophil activation has a pathogenetic role in CFS or a common immunologic background may exist for both atopy and CFS.

Although a higher prevalence of allergy (Steinberg, Pheley, et al., 1996) and delayed-type hypersensitivity (Lloyd et al., 1989, 1992) can be detected in CFS patients, a trial with antihistamine treatment did not provide significant improvement (Steinberg, McNutt, et al., 1996). Other authors, such as Mawle and co-workers (1997), found no significant difference in the incidence of delayed-type hypersensitivity and allergic responses among CFS patients. Baraniuk, Clauw, and Gaumond (1998) and Baraniuk, Clauw, MacDowell-Carneiro, et al. (1998) found that 30 percent of CFS patients had positive skin tests, suggesting the potential for allergic rhinitis complaints, and 46 percent had nonallergic rhinitis and suggested that although atopy may coexist in some CFS subjects, it is unlikely that it plays a causal role in CFS pathogenesis. Borish and co-workers (1998) proposed that in at least a large subgroup of CFS subjects with allergies, the concomitant influences of immune activation brought on by allergic inflammation in an individual with the appropriate psychologic profile may interact to produce the symptoms of CFS. Borok (1998) suggested that food intolerance, in a genetically predisposed group of people, causes symptoms akin to both the major and minor criteria of CFS, and it should be screened for to avoid confusion. On the other hand, some authors have associated CFS with nickel allergy (Marcusson et al., 1999; Regland et al., 2000; Uter, 2000). Although the controversy of atopy and CFS continues, it may be possible that these two conditions share some common denominators that are worth pursuing, particularly in light of the proposed Th2 cytokine predominant pattern.

Chapter 5

Cytokines and Other Soluble Immune Mediators

Stimulated lymphoid cells either express or induce the expression in other cells of a heterogeneous group of soluble mediators that exhibit either effector or regulatory functions. These soluble mediators include cytokines, hormones, and neurotransmitters, which in turn affect immune function and may underlie many of the pathological manifestations seen in CFS (Patarca, Klimas, Sandler, et al., 1995). The studies of cytokines in CFS have been done in the peripheral blood compartment and a review by Vollmer-Conna and coworkers (1998) on the immunopathogenesis of CFS concludes that neuropsychiatric symptoms in CFS patients may be more closely regulated to disordered cytokine production by glial cells within the CNS than to circulating cytokines. The hypothesis that expression of proinflammatory cytokines within the CNS plays a role in the pathogenesis of immunologically mediated fatigue is underscored by the study by Sheng and co-workers (1996) who, using two strains of mice with differential patterns of cytokine expression in response to an injection challenge with *Corynebacterium parvum,* demonstrated that elevated IL-1 and TNF cytokine mRNA expression in the CNS corresponded to development of fatigue. Injection of antibodies specific to either IL-1 or TNF did not alter immunologically induced fatigue, suggesting a lack of involvement of these cytokines produced outside of the CNS. I will nonetheless describe the potential implications of the cytokine imbalances detected in peripheral blood to physiological and psychological functions.

CYTOKINES

The decreased NK cell cytotoxic and lymphoproliferative activities and increased allergic and autoimmune manifestations in CFS would be compatible with the hypothesis that the immune system of affected individuals is biased toward a Th2-type, or humoral immunity-oriented, cytokine pattern (Rook and Zumla, 1997). The factors that could lead to a Th2 shift and to mood changes associated with immunoendocrine changes among CFS patients are unknown. Vaccines and stressful stimuli have been shown to lead to long-term, nonspecific shifts in cytokine balance. Therapeutic regimens that induce a systemic Th1 bias are currently being tested, including repeated stimulation with bacterial antigens or poly (I)-poly (C12U) (Vojdani and Lapp, 1999) and ex vivo activation of lymph node cells (Klimas and Fletcher, 1999).

Proinflammatory and Th1 Cytokines

Interleukin-1 (IL-1) and Soluble IL-1 Receptors

As previously discussed, IL-1 is the term for two distinct cytokines—IL-1alpha and IL-1beta—that share the same cell-surface receptors and biological activities (Dinarello,1991; Platanias and Vogelzang, 1990). One study of CFS patients (Patarca, Lugtendorf, et al., 1994) found elevated levels of serum IL-1alpha but not of plasma IL-1beta in 17 percent of patients studied. When the cohort was examined as to severity of symptoms, it was noted that the top quartile in terms of disability had the highest level of IL-1. Curiously, use of reverse transcriptase-coupled polymerase chain reaction (RT-PCR) revealed IL-1beta, but not IL-1alpha messenger RNA (mRNA) in peripheral blood mononuclear cells (PBMCs) of several CFS patients with highly elevated levels of IL-1alpha. RT-PCR of fractionated cell populations showed that lymphocytes accounted for the IL-1beta mRNA detected in PBMCs. No IL-1 mRNA was apparent in control subjects. The fact that IL-1alpha mRNA was not detectable by RT-PCR in either PBMCs or granulocytes suggests that serum IL-1alpha in CFS patients is probably derived from a source other than peripheral blood cells. Other potential sources are tissue macrophages, endothelial cells, lymph node cells, fibroblasts, central nervous system microglia, astrocytes, and dermal dendritic cells (Dinarello, 1991).

Linde and co-workers (1992) found significantly higher levels of IL-1alpha in CFS and mononucleosis patients, but Lloyd et al. (1992), Peakman et al. (1997) and Rasmussen et al. (1994) found no difference. Five studies, in addition to the one previously described by Patarca, Lugtendorf, et al. (1994), found no difference in the levels of IL-1beta in CFS patients (Linde et al., 1992; Morte et al., 1989; Peakman et al., 1997; Rasmussen et al., 1994; Straus et al., 1989).

The signs and symptoms of CFS, which include fatigue, myalgia, and low-grade fever, are similar to those experienced by patients infused with cytokines such as IL-1. Elevated serum levels of IL-1alpha found in a significant number of CFS patients could underlie several of the clinical symptoms. Interleukin-1 can gain access to the brain through the preoptic nucleus of the hypothalamus, where it induces fever and the release of adrenocorticotropin hormone (ACTH)-releasing factor (Arnason, 1991; Berkenbosch et al., 1987; Besedovsky et al., 1986; Sapolsky et al., 1987), which in turn would lead to release of ACTH and cortisol. The observation that cortisol levels tend to be low in CFS patients regardless of IL-1 alpha levels suggests a role of a defective hypothalamic feedback loop in the pathogenesis of CFS. The presence of such a defect has been documented in Lewis rats, which are particularly susceptible to the induction of a variety of inflammatory and autoimmune diseases and exhibit reduced levels of ACTH-releasing hormone, ACTH, and cortisol in response to IL-1.

Besides its effects on the HPA axis, IL-1 has other effects on the pituitary; it has been shown to augment release of prolactin and growth hormone and to inhibit release of thyrotropin and luteinizing hormone (Bernton et al., 1987; Rettori et al., 1991). The growth hormone deficiency state associated with CFS may also be a reflection of the defect in the hypothalamic feedback loop that renders it inadequately responsive to IL-1.

Interleukin-1 and tumor necrosis factor (TNF) provoke slow-wave sleep when placed in the lateral ventricles of experimental animals (Shoham et al., 1987). The inordinate fatigue, lassitude, and excessive sleepiness associated with CFS (Holmes et al., 1988; Moldovsky, 1989) could well be a consequence of the direct action of these cytokines on neurons. Neurotoxic effects due to chronic overexpression of IL-1alpha and/or beta of S100—a small (10KDa), soluble calcium-binding protein that is synthesized and released by astroglia (Van Eldik and Zimmer, 1987)—have been proposed to underlie progressive neurological degeneration in Alzheimer's disease (Griffin et al., 1989).

IL-1 induces prostaglandin (PGE_2, PGI_2) synthesis by endothelial and smooth muscle cells (Dejana et al., 1987). These substances are potent vasodilators, and IL-1 administration in animals and humans produces significant hypotension. IL-1 has a natriuretic effect (Caverzasio et al., 1987) and may affect plasma volume.

Gulick and colleagues (1989) showed that IL-1 and TNF inhibit beta-adrenergic agonist-mediated cardiac myocyte contractility in cultures and intracellular accumulation of cyclic adenosine monophosphate. Cytokine imbalances may, therefore, also underlie the cardiovascular manifestations of CFS.

Chronic fatigue syndrome is a condition that affects women in disproportionate numbers, and is often exacerbated in the premenstrual period and following physical exertion. Cannon and co-workers (1997) found that isolated peripheral blood mononuclear cells from healthy women, but not from CFS patients, exhibited significant menstrual cycle-related differences in IL-1beta secretion that were related to estradiol and progesterone levels. IL-1Ra secretion for CFS patients was twofold higher than controls during the follicular phase, but luteal-phase levels were similar between groups. In both phases of the menstrual cycle, IL-1sRII release was significantly higher for CFS patients compared to controls. The only changes that might be attributable to exertion occurred in the control subjects during the follicular phase, who exhibited an increase in IL-1beta secretion forty-eight hours after the stress. These results suggest that an abnormality exists in IL-1beta secretion in CFS patients that may be related to altered sensitivity to estradiol and progesterone. Furthermore, the increased release of IL-1Ra and sIL-1RII by cells from CFS patients is consistent with the hypothesis that CFS is associated with chronic, low-level activation of the immune system.

In contrast to these studies, Swanink and co-workers (1996) found no obvious difference in the levels of circulating cytokines, and ex vivo production of IL-1alpha and IL-1 receptor antagonist. Although endotoxin-stimulated ex vivo production of tumor necrosis factor-alpha and IL-beta was significantly lower in CFS, none of the immunologic test results correlated with fatigue severity or psychological well-being scores. Swanink and co-workers (1996) concluded that these immunological tests cannot be used as diagnostic tools in individual CFS patients.

Tumor Necrosis Factors (TNFs) and Soluble TNF Receptors

TNF-alpha and TNF-beta are cytokines produced on lymphoid cell activation (Beutler and Cerami, 1988). Twenty-eight percent of CFS patients studied by Patarca, Lugtendorf, et al. (1994) had elevations in serum levels of TNF-alpha and TNF-beta usually with elevation in serum levels of IL-1 or sIL-2R. TNF-alpha expression in CFS patients is also evident at the mRNA level, which suggests de novo synthesis rather than release of a preformed inducible surface TNF-alpha protein upon activation of monocytes and CD4+ T cells (Kriegler et al., 1988). The levels of spontaneously (unstimulated) produced TNF-alpha by nonadherent lymphocytes were also significantly increased as compared to simultaneously studied matched controls by Gupta and colleagues (1997). Moss et al. (1999) also found elevated levels of TNF-alpha in CFS patients compared to non-CFS controls. TNF-alpha may be associated with CNS pathology because it has been associated with demyelination and may also lead to loss of appetite (Beutler and Cerami, 1988; Wilt et al., 1995). A study by Dreisbach and co-workers (1998) suggests that TNF-alpha may be involved in the pathogenesis of postdialysis fatigue. In contrast to the studies previously discussed, Lloyd et al. (1992) found no difference in the levels of TNF-alpha or -beta in CFS patients, and Rasmussen et al. (1994) and Peakman et al. (1997) found no differences in the levels of TNF-alpha and -beta, respectively. The latter discrepancies are likely due to the fact that TNF levels decrease precipitously if the serum or plasma is not frozen within thirty minutes from collection (Patarca, Sandler, et al., 1995).

TNF-alpha's proinflammatory effects may be mediated by induction of gene expression for neutrophil activating protein-1 and macrophage inflammatory proteins resulting in neutrophil migration and degranulation (Dinarello, 1992). Thus, it is reasonable that TNF elevations may also be associated with markers of macrophage activation such as serum neopterin. Among patients studied at the University of Miami, illness burden scores were significantly positively correlated with elevated TNF-alpha serum levels.

CFS patients have higher levels of sTNF-RI or sCD120a and sTNF-RII or sCD120b (Patarca, Klimas, Sandler, et al., 1995). Higher levels of sTNF-Rs are negatively correlated with NK cell cytotoxic and lymphoproliferative activities in CFS, an observation that is consistent with the activities of these soluble mediators.

Interleukin-2 (IL-2) and Soluble IL-2 Receptor

IL-2, formerly termed "T-cell growth factor," is a glycosylated protein produced by T lymphocytes after mitogenic or antigenic stimulation (Watson and Machizuki, 1980). IL-2 acts as a growth factor (Fletcher and Goldstein, 1987) and promotes proliferation of T cells (Morgan et al., 1976) and, under particular conditions, of B cells and macrophages (Malkovsky et al., 1987; Tsudo et al., 1984). Although serum IL-2 levels were found to be elevated in CFS patients compared with control individuals in one study (Cheney et al., 1989), decreased levels were reported in two other studies (Gold et al., 1990; Kibler et al., 1985), and no difference was reported in three studies (Linde et al., 1992; Patarca, Lugtendorf, et al., 1994; Straus et al., 1989). Rasmussen and co-workers (1994) reported a higher production of IL-2 by stimulated peripheral blood cells from CFS patients as compared to controls. Cheney and co-workers (1989) found no obvious relation between IL-2 serum levels and severity or duration of illness in CFS.

Elevated levels of sIL-2R, a marker of lymphoid cell activation, have been found in a number of pathological conditions including viral infections, autoimmune diseases, and lymphoproliferative and hematological malignancies (Cohen et al., 1990; Pui, 1989). Twelve percent of CFS patients studied by Patarca, Lugtendorf, et al. (1994) had elevated levels of sIL-2R. The latter observation is consistent with the increased proportion of activated T cells and the reduced levels of IL-2 or decreased NK cell cytotoxic activity found in several studies of CFS patients previously discussed. Linde and co-workers (1992) found no elevation in sIL-2R levels in CFS patients.

Interferons (IFNs)

The IFNs comprise a multigenic family with pleiotropic properties and diverse cellular origin. Data from six studies indicate that circulating IFNs are present in 3 percent or less of patients studied (Aoki et al.,

1987; Borysiewicz et al., 1986; Buchwald and Komaroff, 1991; Ho-Yen et al., 1988; Jones et al., 1985; Lloyd et al., 1988; Straus et al., 1985; Vojdani and Lapp, 1999). Peripheral blood cells from children affected by post viral fatigue syndrome produced more IFN-alpha than those from controls. In line with this latter observation, Vojdani and colleagues (1997) found elevated IFN-alpha levels in CFS patients, but Linde et al. (1992) and Straus et al. (1989) found no difference. Fatigue occurs in more than 70 percent of patients treated with IFN-alpha and it may be associated with the development of immune-mediated endocrine diseases, in particular hypothyroidism and hypothalamic-pituitary-adrenal axis-related hormonal deficiencies in these patients (Dalakas et al., 1998; Jones et al., 1998). IFN-alpha therapy-associated fatigue is often the dominant dose-limiting side effect, worsening with continued therapy and accompanied by significant depression. Decreases in mental information processing speeds, verbal memory, and executive functions have also been reported at therapeutic doses of IFN-alpha (Pavol et al., 1995). Although the direct cause of IFN-alpha-induced fatigue is unknown, it is possible that neuromuscular fatigue, similar to that observed in patients with postpolio syndrome, may also be one component of this syndrome. The induction of proinflammatory cytokines observed in patients treated with IFN-alpha is consistent with a possible mechanism of neuromuscular pathology that could manifest as fatigue. A study by Davis and colleagues (1998) also revealed that IFN-alpha/beta is at least partially responsible for the early fatigue induced by polyI:C during prolonged treadmill running in mice.

IFN-gamma is an immunoregulatory substance, enhancing both cellular antigen presentation to lymphocytes (Zlotnick et al., 1983) and NK cell cytotoxicity (Targan and Stebbing, 1982), and causing inhibition of suppressor T-lymphocyte activity (Knop et al., 1982). Two groups have found impaired IFN-gamma production on mitogenic stimulation of peripheral blood mononuclear cells from CFS patients (Klimas et al., 1990; Visser et al., 1998), and one group (Lloyd et al., 1992) found increased production. In contrast with the findings on lymphocyte activation, four groups reported no difference in the levels of circulating IFN-gamma (Linde et al., 1992; Peakman et al., 1997; Straus et al., 1989; Visser et al., 1998). These results are in favor of the Th2 shift described previously, a shift that is not apparent at the level of circulating cytokines.

Th2 Cytokines

Interleukin-4 (IL-4)

Visser and colleagues (1998) reported that although CD4 T cells from CFS patients produce less IFN-gamma than cells from controls, IL-4 production and cell proliferation are comparable. With CD4 T cells from CFS patients (compared with cells from controls), a ten- to twentyfold lower dexamethasone (DEX) concentration was needed to achieve 50 percent inhibition of IL-4 production and proliferation, indicating an increased sensitivity to DEX in CFS patients. In contrast to IL-4, IFN-gamma production in patients and controls was equally sensitive to DEX. A differential sensitivity of cytokines or CD4 T cell subsets to glucocorticoids might explain an altered immunologic function in CFS patients.

IL-4 acts as a growth factor for various types of lymphoid cells, including B, T, and cytotoxic T cells (Paul and Ohara, 1987), and has been shown to be involved in immunoglobulin isotype selection in vivo (Kuehn et al., 1991). Activated T cells are the major source of IL-4 production, but mast cells can also produce it, and IL-4 has been associated with allergic and autoimmune reactions (Paul and Ohara, 1987). It is also noteworthy that many of the effects of IL-4 are antagonized by IFN-gamma, and the decreased production of the latter may underlie a predominance of IL-4 over IFN-gamma effects.

Interleukin-6 (IL-6) and Soluble IL-6 Receptor

The levels of spontaneously produced IL-6 by both adherent monocytes and nonadherent lymphocytes were significantly increased in CFS patients as compared to controls (Gupta et al., 1997, 1999). The abnormality of IL-6 was also observed at mRNA levels. In terms of circulating IL-6, Buchwald and co-workers (1997) found that IL-6 was elevated among febrile CFS patients compared to those without this finding and therefore considered it an epiphenomenon possibly secondary to infection. Chao and co-workers (1990, 1991) also found elevated levels of IL-6 in CFS patients, but five other groups found no difference (Buchwald et al., 1997; Linde et al., 1992; Lloyd et al., 1992; Peakman et al., 1997; See et al., 1997).

Most of the cell types that produce IL-6, do so in response to stimuli such as IL-1 and TNF (Mizel, 1989). Excessive IL-6 production has been associated with polyclonal B-cell activation, resulting in hypegammaglogulinemia and auto antibody production (Van Snick, 1990). As is the case with IL-4, IL-6 may contribute to activation of CD5-bearing B cells, leading to autoimmune manifestations. IL-6 also synergizes with IL-1 in inflammatory reactions and may exacerbate many of the features described previously for IL-1.

Study of cytokine production by stimulated peripheral blood mononuclear cells from patients with a closely related syndrome to CFS, the post–Q-fever fatigue syndrome (QFS) (inappropriate fatigue, myalgia and arthralgia, night sweats, and changes in mood and sleep patterns following about 20 percent of laboratory-proven, acute primary Q-fever cases), showed an accentuated release of IL-6 that was significantly in excess of medians for all four control groups (resolving QFS, acute primary Q-fever without subsequent QFS, healthy Q-fever vaccines, and healthy controls). Levels of induced IL-6 significantly correlated with total symptom scores and scores for other key symptoms (Penttila et al., 1998).

Cannon et al. (1999) found increased IL-6 secretion in CFS patients, which is manifested by chronically elevated plasma alpha2-macroglobulin concentrations. CFS patients have higher levels of sIL-6R (Patarca, Klimas, Garcia, et al., 1995; Patarca, Klimas, Sandler, et al., 1995), and sIL-6R enhances the effects of IL-6.

Interleukin-10 (IL-10)

A study by Gupta and co-workers (1997) revealed that spontaneously produced IL-10 by both adherent monocytes and nonadherent lymphocytes, and by PHA-activated nonadherent monocytes were decreased. IL-10 is part of the Th2-type response.

Tumor Growth Factor-Beta (TGF-Beta)

A study by Bennett and co-workers (1997) found that patients with CFS had significantly higher levels of bioactive TGF-beta levels compared to healthy controls and to patients with various diseases known to be associated with immunologic abnormalities and/or pathologic fatigue: major depression, systemic lupus erythematosus (SLE), and multiple sclerosis (MS) of both the relapsing/remitting (R/R) and the chronic progressive (CP) types.

Other Mediators

Beta-2 Microglobulin

Three studies found elevated levels of beta-2 microglobulin in patients with CFS (Buchwald et al., 1997; Patarca, Klimas, Garcia, et al., 1995; Patarca, Klimas, Sandler, et al., 1995), and one study found no difference (Chao et al., 1990). Beta-2 microglobulin is a marker of immune activation.

Neopterin

Neopterin is a metabolite produced during the utilization of guanosine triphosphate, and increased production of neopterin is associated with macrophage activation by IFN-gamma (Bagasra et al., 1988; Patarca, 1997). Neopterin is a presumed primate homolog of nitric oxide, which activated guanylate cyclase, and is involved in the neurotransmission, vasodilation, neurotoxicity, inhibition of platelet aggregation, antiproliferative action of cytokines, and reduction of oxidative stress (Fuchs et al., 1994, 1995). Neopterin derivatives belong to the cytotoxic arsenal of the activated human macrophage, and in high doses, increase oxidative stress through enhancement of radical-mediated effector functions and programmed cell death by TNF-alpha, although it has an opposite effect at low doses (Baier-Bitterlich et al., 1995; Fuchs et al., 1994, 1995). Buchwald et al. (1997) and Chao et al. (1990, 1991) found elevated levels of neopterin in CFS patients, and Linde et al. (1992) and Patarca, Lugtendorf, et al. (1994) found no difference. A report of nine CFS cases showed significantly elevated serum neopterin levels in association with high cognitive difficulty scale (CDS) scores (Lugtendorf, Antoni, et al., 1995; Lugtendorf, Klimas, et al., 1995), and neopterin levels have been shown to correlate with levels of many other mediators that have been found to be dysregulated in CFS, including members of the TNF family (Buchwald et al., 1997; Patarca, Lugtendorf, et al., 1994; Patarca, Klimas, Garcia, et al., 1995; Patarca, Klimas, Sandler, et al., 1995). In terms of neurotoxicity, serum neopterin and tryptophan concentrations correlate among cancer and AIDS patients, an observation that can be accounted for by activity of indoleamine 2,3-dioxygenase, a tryptophan-degrading enzyme (Fuchs et al., 1990; Iwagaki et al., 1995). The latter enzyme also converts L-tryptophan to L-kynurenine, kynurenic acid, and quinolinic acid (QUIN). QUIN is a neurotoxic metabolite that accumulates within the CNS following immune activation and is also a sensitive marker for the presence of immune activation within the CNS (Heyes et al., 1995; Saito, 1995; Shaskan et al., 1992). Direct conversion of L-tryptophan into QUIN by brain tissue occurs in conditions of CNS inflammation, but not by normal brain tissue. Macrophage infiltrates, and perhaps microglia, are important sources of QUIN, an observation that is consistent with the results of inoculation of poliovirus directly into the spinal cord of rhesus macaque monkey, resulting in increased CSF levels of both QUIN and neopterin (Andondonskaja-Renz and Zeitler, 1984; Heyes et al., 1995). Elevated serum levels of neopterin correlate with the presence of brain lesions and with neurologic and psychiatric symptoms in patients with AIDS dementia complex (Lutgendorf, Klimas, et al., 1995; Sonnerborg et al., 1990). It is worth noting in this context that Buchwald and colleagues (1992) found subcortical lesions consistent with edema and demyelination by magnetic resonance scans in 78 percent of CFS patients as compared to 20 percent of controls.

Soluble CD8 (sCD8)

Linde and co-workers (1992) found no elevation of sCD8 in CFS patients.

Soluble ICAM-1 (sICAM-1)

Patarca, Klimas, Garcia, et al. (1995) and Patarca, Klimas, Sandler, et al. (1995) found higher levels of sICAM-1 in CFS patients, an observation that is consistent with the higher expresion of ICAM-1 in monocytes of CFS patients reported by Gupta and Vayuvegula (1991).

IMMUNOGLOBULINS

Spontaneous and mitogen-induced immunoglobulin synthesis is depressed in 10 percent of patients with CFS (Borysiewicz et al., 1986; Hamblin et al., 1983; Tosato et al., 1985). The latter decrease may be a result of an increased T-cell suppression of immunoglobulin synthesis, because a similar effect is obtained in vitro when using normal allogeneic B cells (Tosato et al., 1985). This inhibitory effect may also account for the reported difficulty in establishing spontaneous outgrowth of EBV-transformed B-cell lines from cells from CFS patients (Buchwald and Komaroff, 1991; Straus et al., 1985; Tosato et al., 1985). The depletion of the CD4+CD45RA+ lymphocyte subset in the studies by Klimas et al. (1990) and Franco et al. (1987), may be associated with alteration in B-cell regulation.

In twelve studies, CFS patients were found to have decreased amounts of immunoglobulins of the G, A, M, or D classes (Buchwald and Komaroff, 1991; DuBois, 1986; Hilgers and Frank, 1996; Jones et al., 1985; Lloyd et al., 1989; Rasmussen et al., 1994; Read et al., 1988; Roubalova et al., 1988; Salit, 1985; Straus et al., 1985; Tosato et al., 1985; Wakefield et al., 1990); in five studies no difference was found (Gupta and Vayuvegula, 1991; Lloyd et al., 1992; Mawle et al., 1997; Natelson et al., 1998; Peakman et al., 1997); and in one study IgG levels were elevated and IgA levels were normal (Bates et al., 1995). IgG subclass deficiency, particularly of the opsonins IgG1 or IgG3, can be demonstrated in a substantial percentage of CFS patients (Klimas et al., 1990; Komaroff et al., 1988; Linde et al., 1988; Lloyd et al., 1989; Read et al., 1988; Wakefield et al., 1990). For a subset of these, immunoglobulin replacement therapy may be beneficial (Lloyd et al., 1990; Peterson et al., 1990; Rowe, 1997; Straus, 1990), albeit controversial (Straus, 1990; Vollmer-Conna et al., 1997). Bennett and co-workers (1996) also failed to find immunoglobulin subclass deficiencies in CFS patients.

AUTOANTIBODIES

Konstantinov and colleagues (1996) found that approximately 52 percent of sera from CFS patients react with nuclear envelope antigens. Some sera immunoprecipitated nuclear envelope protein lamin B1, an observation that underscores an autoimmune component in CFS (Poteliakhoff, 1998). Von Mikecz and colleagues (1997) found a high frequency (83 percent) of autoantibodies to insoluble cellular antigens (vimentin and lamin B1) in CFS, a unique feature that might help to distinguish CFS from other rheumatic autoimmune diseases. Another finding that underscores a possible autoimmune etiology is the significant association between CFS and the presence of HLA-DQ3 reported by Keller and colleagues (1994).

The presence of rheumatoid factor (Jones et al., 1985; Jones and Straus, 1987; Jones, 1991; Kaslow et al., 1989; Prieto et al., 1989; Roubalova et al., 1988; Straus et al., 1985; Tobi et al., 1982); antinuclear antibodies (Bates et al., 1995; Gold et al., 1990; Jones et al., 1985; Jones and Straus, 1987; Jones, 1991; Nishikai and Kosaka, 1997; Prieto et al., 1989; Salit, 1985; Straus et al., 1985; Tobi et al., 1982; von Mikecz et al., 1997); antithyroid antibodies (Behan et al., 1985; Tobi et al., 1982; Weinstein, 1987); antismooth-muscle antibodies (Behan et al., 1985); antiphospholipid antibodies (Berg et al., 1999); anti-p80 coilin antibodies (Onouchi et al., 1999); antigliadin, cold agglutinins; cryoglobulins; and false serological positivity for syphilis (Behan et al., 1985; Straus et al., 1985) have also been reported. No circulating antimuscle and anti-CNS antibodies were found in ten CFS patients (Plioplys, 1997), and Rasmussen and co-workers (1994) found no significant differences in the number of positive tests for auto-antibodies in CFS patients.

CIRCULATING IMMUNE COMPLEXES

Elevated levels of immune complexes have been reported in four studies (Bates et al., 1995; Behan et al., 1985; Borysiewicz et al., 1986; Straus et al., 1985), and the studies by Natelson et al. (1998) and Mawle et al. (1997) revealed no abnormality in the level of circulating immune complexes (i.e., Raji cell and C1q binding). Depressed levels of complement have also been reported in up to 25 percent of patients (Behan et al., 1985; Borysiewicz et al., 1986; Mawle et al., 1997; Natelson et al., 1998; Straus et al., 1985). Buchwald and co-workers (1997) found elevated levels of C-reactive protein among CFS patients.

Chapter 6

Potential Infectious and Autoimmune Etiologies for Chronic Fatigue Syndrome

INFECTIOUS AGENTS AS POSSIBLE DIRECT CAUSES OF CFS

After having reviewed the immunological changes that have been associated with CFS, this chapter addresses several of their possible causes. The links between immune, endocrine, and nervous system abnormalities were discussed in Chapter 2. This chapter focuses on the links between infectious diseases, autoimmunity, and CFS.

Viruses

Several families of viruses have been studied in association with CFS, including enteroviruses, herpesviruses, stealth viruses, retroviruses, lentiviruses, parvovirus B19, Ross River virus, and Borna disease virus. There are also many historical accounts of diseases of presumed viral etiology that present similar to CFS, including George Reinhold Forster's description of the Tapanui flu and the documentation of Akureyri or Iceland disease (Lindal et al., 1997; St. George, 1996). It has also been proposed that reactivation of certain viruses may play a role in the pathophysiology of CFS, but may not be its primary cause.

Enteroviruses

Enteroviruses (Coxsackie virus A and B, echovirus, poliovirus) belong to a group of small RNA viruses, picornavirus, which are widespread in nature. Enteroviruses cause a number of well-known diseases and symptoms in humans, from subclinical infections and the common cold to poliomyelitis with paralysis. Serologic and molecular biology techniques have demonstrated that enteroviral genomes, in certain situations, persist after the primary infection, which is often silent. Persistent enteroviral infection or recurrent infections and/or virus-stimulated autoimmunity might contribute to the development of diseases with hitherto unexplained pathogenesis, such as post-polio syndrome, dilated cardiomyopathy, juvenile (type 1) diabetes, and possibly some cases diagnosed as CFS (Archard et al., 1988; Fohlman et al., 1997; Galbraith et al., 1997; Hill, 1996; Miller et al., 1991). Several studies have failed to document persistent enteroviral infections in CFS (Buchwald, Ashley, et al., 1996; Lindh et al., 1996; McArdle et al., 1996).

Herpesviruses

Herpesviruses (Epstein-Barr virus, cytomegalovirus, human herpesvirus types 6 and 7, herpes simplex virus types 1 and 2) have been associated with CFS. For instance, reactivation/replication of a latent herpesvirus (such as Epstein-Barr virus) could modulate the immune system to induce CFS (Glaser and Kiecolt-Glaser, 1998; Glaser et al., 1999; Hellinger et al., 1988; Jones et al., 1985). In this respect, serologically proven acute infectious illness secondary to Epstein-Barr virus (EBV) is associated with a range of nonspecific somatic and psychological symptoms, particularly fatigue and malaise rather than anxiety and depression (Bennett et al., 1998). Although improvement in several symptoms occurs rapidly, fatigue commonly remains a prominent complaint at four weeks, and resolution of fatigue is associated with improvement in cell-mediated immunity. A prospective cohort study of 250 primary care patients also revealed a higher incidence and longer duration of an acute fatigue syndrome, and a higher prevalence of CFS, after glandular fever as compared to after an ordinary upper-respiratory tract infection (White et al., 1998). In another study, anti-EBV titers were higher among CFS patients and were associated with being more symptomatic (Schmaling and Jones, 1996). Ablashi et al. (2000) also proposed that HHV-6 reactivation plays a role in the pathogenesis of CFS and multiple sclerosis. However, testing of 548 chronically fatigued individuals, including patients with CFS, for antibodies to thirteen viruses (herpes simplex virus 1 and 2, rubella, adenovirus, human herpesvirus 6, Epstein-Barr virus, cytomegalovirus, and Coxsackie B virus types 1 through 6) in patients found no consistent differences in any of the seroprevalences compared with controls (Buchwald, Ashley, et al., 1996). A study by Wallace et al. (1999) reached a similar conclusion.

Some studies suggest an association between human herpesvirus-6 (HHV-6) (*Roseolovirus* genus of the betaherpesvirus subfamily) and CFS (Braun et al., 1997; Cuende et al., 1997; Levy et al., 1990; Marsh et al., 1996). One study found that a high proportion of CFS patients (50 percent by antibody testing and up to 80 percent by nested-PCR detection of viral DNA but not RNA) were infected with HHV-6 but with low viral load. The latter results do not support HHV-6 reactivation in CFS patients (Cuende et al., 1997). Other studies have addressed a possible association between HHV-7 and CFS. Use of the supernatant fluid from HHV-7 infected cells as antigen in immunoassays yielded high and low HHV-7 antibody in sera from chronic fatigue patients and healthy donors as controls, respectively (Ablashi et al., 1998).

Stealth Viruses

Cloned DNA obtained from the culture of an African green monkey simian cytomegalovirus-derived stealth virus contains multiple discrete regions of significant sequence homology to portions of known human cellular genes (Martin, 1998, 1999). The stealth virus has also been cultured from several CFS patient and a cytopathic stealth virus was also cultured from the cerebrospinal fluid of a nurse with CFS. The findings lend support to the possibility of replicative RNA forms of certain stealth viruses (Martin, 1997). Review of the clinical histories and brain biopsy findings of three patients with severe stealth virus encephalopathy showed that the patients initially developed symptoms consistent with CFS (Martin, 1996a,b). One patient has remained in a vegetative state for several years, and the other two patients have shown significant, although incomplete, recovery. Histological and electron-microscopic studies revealed vacuolated cells with distorted nuclei and various cytoplasmic inclusions suggestive of incomplete viral expression. There was no significant inflammatory response. Viral cultures provided further evidence of stealth viral infections occurring in these patients (Martin, 1996b). Partial sequencing of stealth virus segments isolated from a CFS patient revealed a fragmented genome and sequence microheterogeneity, observations that suggest that both the processivity and the fidelity of replication of the viral genome are defective (Martin, 1996a). An unstable viral genome may provide a potential mechanism of recovery from stealth viral illness.

Retroviruses

Some studies (DeFreitas et al., 1991; Gunn et al., 1997) looked into a possible link between retroviruses and CFS, but no conclusive evidence has been garnered.

Lentiviruses

Although structures consistent in size, shape, and character with various stages of a lentivirus replicative cycle were observed by electron microscopy in twelve-day peripheral-blood lymphocyte cultures from ten of seventeen CFS patients and not in controls, attempts to identify a lymphoid phenotype containing these structures failed and the results of reverse-transcriptase assay of culture supernatant fluids were equivocal (Holmes et al., 1997).

Parvovirus B19

The spectrum of disease caused by parvovirus B19 has been expanding in recent years because of improved and more sensitive methods of detection. There is evidence to suggest that chronic infection occurs in patients who are not detectably immunosuppressed. A young woman with recurrent fever and a syndrome indistinguishable from CFS was found to have persistent parvovirus B19 viremia, which was detectable by polymerase chain reaction despite the presence of IgM and IgG antibodies to parvovirus B19 (Jacobson et al., 1997). Testing of samples from this patient suggested that in some low viremic states parvovirus B19 DNA is detectable by nested PCR in plasma but not in serum. The patient's fever resolved with the administration of intravenous immunoglobulin.

Ross River Virus

A prospective investigation revealed that serologically proven acute infectious illness due to Ross River virus is associated with a range of nonspecific somatic and psychological symptoms, particularly fatigue and malaise rather than anxiety and depression (Bennett et al., 1998). Although improvement in several symptoms occurs rapidly, fatigue commonly remains a prominent complaint at four weeks. Resolution of fatigue is associated with improvement in cell-mediated immunity as measured by delayed-type hypersensitivity skin responses.

Borna Disease Virus

Borna disease virus (BDV) is a neurotropic, nonsegmented, negative-sense single-strand RNA virus (Nowotny and Kolodziejek, 2000). Natural infection with this virus has been reported to occur in horses and sheep. Recent epidemiological data suggest that BDV may be closely associated with neuropsychiatric disease (depression and schizophrenia) in humans (Bode et al., 1993; Kitani et al., 1996; Levine, 1999; Nakaya et al., 1996, 1997; Salvatore et al., 1998; Sauder et al., 1996; Stitz et al., 1993; Yamaguchi et al., 1999). In Japanese patients with CFS, the prevalence of BDV infection is up to 34 percent. Furthermore, anti-BDV antibodies and BDV RNA were detected in a family cluster with CFS. Nakaya et al. (1997) focused on BDV infection in two family clusters of CFS patients. All members, except for the elder son in one family and the father and the son in the second family, were diagnosed with CFS. All the family members with CFS were infected with BDV, as evidenced by the presence of antibodies to viral p40, p24 and/or gp18, and BDV p24 RNA in peripheral blood mononuclear cells. The healthy members, except for the father of the second family who was positive for antibody to p24, were all negative by both assays. These results suggest that BDV or a related agent may contribute to or initiate CFS, although the single etiologic role of BDV is unlikely (Bode et al., 1993; Kitani et al., 1996; Levine, 1999; Nakaya et al., 1996, 1997; Salvatore et al., 1998; Sauder et al., 1996; Stitz et al., 1993). In this respect, a Swedish study found no specific immunoreactivity to BDV proteins in sera from 169 patients or 62 controls (Evengard et al., 1999). Moreover, no BDV- or P-gene transcripts were found through RT-PCR analysis of PBMCs from eighteen patients with severe CFS.

Bacteria

Borrelia

Despite antibiotic treatment, a sequela of Lyme disease may be a post-Lyme disease syndrome (PLS), which is characterized by persistent arthralgia, fatigue, and neurocognitive impairment (Bujak et al., 1996; Diamantis, 1996; Ellenbogen, 1997; Ravdin et al., 1996). Although patients with CFS and PLS share many features, including symptoms of severe fatigue and cognitive impairment, patients with PLS show greater cognitive deficits than patients with CFS compared with healthy controls. This is particularly apparent among patients with PLS without premorbid psychiatric illness (Gaudino et al., 1997). Schutzer and Natelson (1999) pointed out that CFS patients lacking antecedent signs of Lyme disease—erythema migrans, Bell's palsy, or large joint arthritis—are not likely to have laboratory evidence of *Borrelia* infection. Treib et al. (2000) conducted a prospective double-blind study of 156 healthy young males testing for *Borrelia* antibodies. Seropositive subjects who had never suffered from clinically manifest Lyme borreliosis or neuroborreliosis showed significantly more often chronic fatigue and malaise than seronegative recruits. Treib et al. (2000) therefore proposed that it is worth examining whether an antibiotic therapy should be considered in patients with chronic fatigue syndrome and positive *Borrelia* serology.

Chlamydia

Some authors have proposed a link between *Chlamydia* bacteria and CFS (Bottero, 2000; Chia and Chia, 1999).

Mycoplasma

Multiplex polymerase chain reaction analysis to detect the presence of *Mycoplasma* genus DNA sequences in 100 CFS patients revealed that 52 percent were infected with *Mycoplasma* genus as compared to 15 percent of healthy individuals. *Mycoplasma fermentans, hominis,* and *penetrans* were detected in 32, 9, and 6 percent of the CFS patients, but only in 8, 3, and 2 percent of the healthy control subjects, respectively (Choppa et al., 1998). An analysis of studies based on the use of forensic polymerase chain reaction or polymerase chain reaction found that 52 to 63 percent of CFS/FMS patients (n ~1000) had mycoplasmal infections, whereas 9 to 15 percent of controls (n ~450) tested positive (Choppa et al., 1998; Nicolson et al., 1998, 2000; Vojdani et al., 1998; Vojdani and Franco, 1999). Nasralla et al. (1999) found multiple mycoplasmal infections by polymerase chain reaction in forty-eight of ninety-one CFS/fibromyalgia patients with a positive serological test for mycoplasmal infection, with double infections being detected in 30.8 percent and triple infections in 22 percent, but only when one of the species was *Mycoplasma pneumoniae* or *Mycoplasma fermentans*. Patients infected with more than one mycoplasmal species generally had a longer history of illness, suggesting that they may have contracted additional mycoplasmal infections with time (Nasralla et al., 1999).

Rickettsiae

Several links have been proposed since 1991 between CFS and chronic Rickettsial infection (Jadin, 1962, 1999, 2000), including:

1. CFS and Rickettsial infection present with a similar symptomatology.
2. CFS was reported in Incline, Nevada, in 1984 (Mauff and Gon, 1991) and developed into epidemic proportions. Rocky Mountain spotted fever originated from the same place in 1916 (Jadin, 1953). Drury described the spirochete *Borrelia duttoni*, in 1702 as causing recurrent Malgach fever. In 1975, *Borrelia burgdorferi* was found in Connecticut, giving birth to a new name, Lyme disease.
3. A link has been established between CFS and Florence Nightingale (Hennessy, 1994), who worked surrounded by lice, fleas, and ticks during the Crimean war. Soldiers were presenting with epidemic typhus, the common disease of wars, regularly reported since the time of Hannibal.
4. Lymphocyte studies conducted on sheep with tickborne diseases (Woldehiwe, 1991), CFS patients, and patients with Q-fever endocarditis (Drancourt, 1990) have shown similar results.
5. CFS was proposed to overlap with post–Q-fever syndrome (Marmion et al., 1996).

Post–Q-fever fatigue syndrome (QFS) is characterized by inappropriate fatigue, myalgia and arthralgia, night sweats, and changes in mood and sleep patterns following about 20 percent of laboratory-proven, acute primary Q-fever cases, a condition caused by *Coxiella burnetti* (Ayres et al., 1998; Bennett et al., 1998; Marmion et al., 1996). The condition is associated with high levels of interleukin-6, and although improvement in several symptoms occurs rapidly, resolution of fatigue takes longer and it is associated with improvement in cell-mediated immunity as measured by delayed-type hypersensitivity skin responses (Penttila et al., 1998). The recovery rate associated with treatment of CFS patients with tetracyclines by several practitioners is 84 to 96 percent (Bottero, 2000; Jadin, 1998; Tarbleton, 1995).

Yersinia

A study based on the detection of antibodies to various *Yersinia* outer membrane proteins (YOPs) in serum samples from eighty-eight CFS patients and seventy-seven healthy age- and gender-matched controls concluded that *Yersinia enterocolitica* is unlikely to play a major role in the etiology of CFS (Swanink et al., 1998).

Fungi

Sorenson (1999) places chronic fatigue syndrome among the diseases associated with inhalation of fungal spores.

AUTOIMMUNITY AND CFS: INFECTIOUS AGENTS AS POSSIBLE INDIRECT CAUSES OF CFS

Another etiological hypothesis for CFS is that an acute microbial infection triggers an autoimmune response, i.e., when the body mounts an attack against the virus, it selects the production of immuno-globulins that can also recognize and attack the body itself. This happens because of what is termed "molecular mimicry" (Atkinson et al., 1994; Banki et al., 1992; Blick et al., 1990; Ciampolillo et al., 1989; Dang et al., 1991; Gama Sosa et al., 1997; Garry et al., 1990; Jones and Armstrong, 1995; Lagaye et al., 1992; Perl et al., 1991; Silvestris et al., 1995; Talal, Dauphinée, et al., 1990; Talal, Garry, et al., 1990; Tian et al., 1994; Trujillo et al., 1993). The portions of the microbe that the antibodies recognize somehow resemble those of proteins that normally constitute the human body. The evidence for autoimmunity in CFS comes from several sources. One research team found that approximately 52 percent of sera from CFS patients react with nuclear envelope antigens (Konstantinov et al., 1996). Some sera from CFS patients immunoprecipitated the nuclear envelope protein lamin B1 (Poteliakhoff, 1998). Another report documented a high frequency (83 percent) of auto antibodies to insoluble cellular antigens (vimentin and lamin B1) in CFS, a unique feature that might help to distinguish CFS from other rheumatic autoimmune diseases (von Mikecz et al., 1997). The possible autoimmune etiology of CFS is further underscored by preliminary evidence for an association between CFS and the presence of HLA-DQ3 (Keller et al., 1994).

Several studies have documented the presence in CFS patients of rheumatoid factor (Jones, 1991; Jones and Straus, 1987; Kaslow et al., 1989; Prieto et al., 1989; Salit, 1985; Straus et al., 1985; Tobi et al., 1982); antinuclear antibodies (Bates et al., 1995; Keller et al., 1994; Jones, 1991; Jones and Straus, 1987; Kaslow et al., 1989; Poteliakhoff, 1998; Prieto et al., 1989; Salit, 1985; Straus et al., 1985; Tobi et al., 1982); antithyroid antibodies (Behan et al., 1985; Tobi et al., 1982; Weinstein, 1987); anti–smooth-muscle antibodies (Behan et al., 1985); antiphospholipid antibodies (Berg et al., 1999); anti-p80 coilin antibodies (Onouchi et al., 1999); antigliadin, cold agglutinins; cryoglobulins; and false serological positivity for syphilis (Behan et al., 1985; Straus et al., 1985). No circulating antimuscle and anti-CNS antibodies were found in ten CFS patients (Plioplys, 1997), and one group found no significant differences in the number of positive tests for auto antibodies in CFS patients (Rasmussen et al., 1994).

One team found that among children who chronically complain of nonspecific symptoms such as headache, fatigue, abdominal pain, and low-grade fever, those who were antinuclear antibody (ANA) positive tended to have general fatigue and low-grade fever, although gastrointestinal problems such as abdominal pain and diarrhea and orthostatic dysregulation symptoms were commonly seen in ANA-negative patients (Itoh et al., 1997). Children who were unable to go to school more than one day a week were seen significantly more among ANA-positive patients than among ANA-negative patients. Based on these observations, Itoh and colleagues concluded that autoimmunity may play a role in childhood chronic nonspecific symptoms and proposed a new disease entity: the autoimmune fatigue syndrome in children.

The features shared between CFS and autoimmune diseases may complicate diagnosis. For instance, three cases of dermatomyositis had been erroneously diagnosed as CFS because of the presence of elevated titers of serum Epstein-Barr virus antibodies (Fiore et al., 1997). In one study, one-third of CFS patients with sicca symptoms fulfilled the diagnostic criteria for Sjoegren's syndrome, but they were "seronegative," differing from the ordinary primary Sjoegren's syndrome (Nishikai et al., 1996). An additional confounding feature is that patients with primary Sjoegren's syndrome report more fatigue than healthy controls on all the dimensions of the Multidimensional Fatigue Inventory and, when controlling for depression, significant differences remain on the dimensions of general fatigue, physical fatigue, and reduced activity (Barendregt et al., 1998). The negative correlation between levels of noradrenaline and general fatigue in patients with primary Sjoegren's syndrome may imply the involvement of the autonomic nervous system in the chronic fatigue reported in this syndrome (Asim and Turney, 1997; Barendregt et al., 1998). Although fatigue in patients with systemic lupus erythematosus (SLE) does not correlate with disease activity, it is correlated with fibromyalgia, depression, and lower overall health status (Wang et al., 1998). Fatigue is also a major symptom in patients with ankylosing spondylitis and, unlike SLE, it is more likely to occur with active disease but it may occur as a lone symptom (Jones et al., 1996). Fatigue is also common in osteoarthritis and rheumatoid arthritis, associates with measures of distress, and is a predictor of work dysfunction and overall health status (Wolfe et al., 1996). Several studies have reported that rheumatoid arthritis-related fatigue is strongly associated with psychosocial variables, apart from disease activity per se (Huyser et al., 1998; Riemsma et al., 1998). Fatigue is associated to a large extent with pain; self-efficacy toward coping with disease, asking for help, and problematic social support; and female gender. One study found large individual differences in variation of pain and fatigue among rheumatoid arthritis patients (Stone et al., 1997). Stressors were associated with increased pain but not fatigue. Subjects with poor sleep had higher levels of pain and fatigue. Diurnal cycles of pain and fatigue were found yet were observed in only some patients.

Studies of lymph node cells from CFS patients (Fletcher et al., 2000) also reveal changes in phenotypic distributions that are similar to those found in several autoimmune diseases. In this respect, although Tedla et al. (1999) reported that the majority of the CD4+ and CD8+ T lymphocytes obtained from both lymph nodes and peripheral blood of control subjects were immunologically naive (CD45RA+), Fletcher et al. (2000) found that in both lymph nodes and peripheral blood of CFS patients a greater proportion of lymphocytes had the "memory" phenotype (CD45RO+). Klimas et al. (1990) had previously reported a decreased proportion of CD4+CD45RA+ cells in the peripheral blood compartment of CFS patients. CD4+CD45RA+ lymphocytes are associated with suppressor/cytotoxic cell induction (Morimoto et al., 1985), and CD45RA+ lymphocytes preferentially home into lymph nodes (Mackay et al., 1990; Mackay, 1992; Westemann and Pabst, 1996). Although one group (Natelson et al., 1998) found no significant change in the proportions of CD4+ CD45RA+ and CD4+CD45RO+ cells in CFS patients, another group also described a decrease in the number of CD4+CD45RA+ lymphocytes in two patients with severe, chronic, active Epstein-Barr virus (EBV) infection (Franco et al., 1987). One of the two patients showed a persistent diminished number of cells despite clinical improvement with IL-2 treatment. Besides herpesviruses as possible etiological agents for CFS, other authors have proposed that CFS is an autoimmune disease and several publications have associated decreased proportions in the CD45RA+ subset of lymphocytes with autoimmune diseases (i.e., systemic lupus erythematosus, procainamide-induced lupus, rheumatoid arthritis, Sjoegren's syndrome, and multiple sclerosis) (Alpert et al., 1987; Emery et al., 1987; Klimas, Morgan, et al., 1992; Morimoto et al., 1985; Sato et al., 1987; Sobel et al., 1988).

Chapter 7

The Th1/Th2 Imbalance Paradigm in Chronic Fatigue Syndrome

Chronic fatigue syndrome is characterized by debilitating fatigue that is not attributable to known clinical conditions, that has lasted for more than six months, that has reduced the activity level of a previously healthy person by more than 50 percent, and that has been accompanied by flulike symptoms (e.g., pharyngitis, adenopathy, low-grade fever, myalgia, arthralgia, headache) and neuropsychological manifestations (e.g., difficulty concentrating, exercise intolerance, and sleep disturbances) (Buchwald et al., 1992; Fukuda et al., 1994; Holmes et al., 1988; Klimas and Fletcher, 1995; Lutgendorf, Antoni, et al., 1995; Lutgendorf, Klimas, et al., 1995; Millon et al., 1989; Patarca, 2000).

Although syndromes are clusters of nonchance associations, and the components of a syndrome can be generally related to a common element, the cause of CFS still remains to be determined. CFS is frequently of sudden onset. Possible precipitating factors include infections, psychiatric trauma, and exposure to toxins (Ablashi et al., 1995; Chester and Levine, 1994; Klimas, Morgan, et al., 1992; Patarca, 2000). Even among those who favor a microbial etiology for CFS, it is not yet clear whether CFS is a consequence of a chronic microbial infection or of an acute microbial infection that resolves, but whose sequel in the form of autoimmunity or other manifestations is responsible for the pathology seen. Microbial reactivation may also play a causal or perpetuating role in disease manifestation.

A review of the literature on the immunology of CFS reveals that people who have chronic fatigue syndrome have two basic problems with immune function, which have been documented by most research groups: (1) immune activation, as demonstrated by elevation of activated T lymphocytes, including cytotoxic T cells, as well as elevations of circulating cytokines; and (2) poor cellular function, with low natural killer cell cytotoxicity (NKCC), poor lymphocyte response to mitogens in culture, and frequent immunoglobulin deficiencies, most often IgG1 and IgG3. These findings have a waxing and waning temporal pattern that is consistent with episodic immune dysfunction (with predominance of so-called T-helper type 2 and proinflammatory cytokines and low NKCC and lymphoproliferation) that can be associated as cause or effect of the physiological and psychological function derangement and/or activation of latent viruses or other pathogens. The interplay of these factors can account for the perpetuation of disease with remission/exacerbation cycles. Therapeutic intervention aimed at induction of a more favorable cytokine expression pattern and immune status is discussed.

One of the models of CFS holds that the interaction of psychological factors (distress associated with either CFS-related symptoms or other stressful life events) and immunologic dysfunction (indicated in signs of chronic overactivation with cytokine abnormalities) contribute to: (a) CFS-related physical symptoms (e.g., fatigue, joint pain, cognitive difficulties, fever) and increases in illness burden; and (b) dysfunction in the immune system's ability to survey viruses including latent herpesviruses (indicated in impaired NKCC). As discussed previously, there is a decrease in the ratio of type 1/type 2 cytokines produced by lymphocytes in vitro following mitogen stimulation in CFS patients. This type of dysfunction should be expected to result in impaired immune surveillance associated with cytotoxic lymphocytes. For example, Cohen et al. (1991) found an association between psychosocial stressors, immunomodulation, and the incidence and progression of rhinovirus infections in healthy normals. Here, the rates of respiratory infections and clinical colds increased in a dose-response fashion with increases in psychological stress across all five of the cold viruses studied. If viruses related to upper-respiratory tract infections (URIs) are not well controlled by immune surveillance mechanisms (e.g., NKCC) in CFS patients who are exposed to stressors, then patients may suffer more frequent and protracted URIs that are accompanied by prolonged elevations in proinflammatory cytokines. Stress-associated reactivation of latent herpesviruses may also play a role in modulating the production of cytokines that underlie CFS symptom exacerbations (Glaser et al., 1999; Glaser and Kiecolt-Glaser, 1998). Alternatively, distress increases may more directly influence cytokine dysregulation by way of neuroendocrine changes, which in turn intensify physical symptoms. Equally important, for all of the possible paths, further increases in distress as a "reaction" to mounting symptoms create a vicious cycle. Such a recursive system may act as a positive feedback loop thereby accounting for the chronic nature of CFS and its refraction to interventions that focus solely on symptom reduction.

The conceptual model for CFS previously discussed was supported by data showing that distress levels in response to the stressor Hurricane Andrew were positively correlated with: alterations in NK cells and elevated (compared to prestorm values) circulating levels of the cytokines; exacerbation in CFS symptoms; and increases in Sickness Impact Profile (SIP)-based illness burden scores among CFS patients (Lutgendorf, Antoni, et al., 1995; Lutgendorf, Klimas, et al., 1995). This study found that CFS patients living in a hurricane exposure area (Dade County) had significantly greater severity of CFS symptom relapses (using clinician-rated fatigue levels and ability to engage in work-related activities), and significantly greater increases in illness burden as compared to age- and gender-matched CFS patients from the same clinical practice living in an adjacent geographical region that was not in the storm's path, Broward/Palm Beach County. This study also found that pre–post-hurricane NKCC changes were associated with pre–post-storm symptom severity changes including cognitive symptoms, muscle weakness, and muscle pain. These data suggested that stressor-induced decrements in NKCC were associated with greater increases in the severity of cognitive difficulties, muscle weakness, and pain symptoms. A final regression analysis on NKCC indicated that appraisals in greater storm impact and low social support predicted the greatest pre–post-storm decrements in NKCC. Greater optimism and social support provisions were also associated with less elevations in TNF-alpha among storm victims.

The increased autoimmune manifestations in CFS, along with the decreased natural killer cell cytotoxic and lymphoproliferative activities, would be compatible with the hypothesis that the immune systems of affected individuals are biased toward a T-helper (Th)2 type, or humoral immunity (antibody producing)-oriented cytokine expression pattern, over a Th1 type, or cellular mediated (natural killer cell and macrophage activating) immunity-oriented one. Potent immunogens can have systemic long-lasting, nonspecific effects on the nature of the immune response to unrelated antigens. In particular, vaccinations or infections can exert a systemic effect, and nonspecifically increase or reduce the Th1/Th2 cytokine balance of the response to other unrelated antigens (Shaheen et al., 1996) and affect (positively or negatively) survival from unrelated diseases (Aaby, 1995; Aaby et al., 1995).

Based on the fact that Gulf War personnel were given multiple Th2-type response-inducing vaccinations, Rook, Stanford, and Zumla, in international published patent number WO-09826790, presented the hypothesis that Gulf War syndrome represents a special case of CFS, where the Th-2 inducing stimuli can be identified. Rook and colleagues pointed out that induction of a systemic Th2 switch is underscored by four features of the vaccination protocol used for the Gulf War troops.

First, pertussis was used as an adjuvant in British troops in the Persian Gulf and its adjuvanticity is potently Th2-type response-inducing (Mu and Sewell, 1993; Ramiya et al., 1996; Smit et al., 1996). This property of pertussis has recently led to discussion of the possibility that its use in children contributes to the contemporary increased prevalence of atopy (Nilsson et al., 1996; Odent et al., 1994).

Second, Gulf War troops were given Th2-inducing immunogens against plague, anthrax, typhoid, tetanus, and cholera. Such a cumulatively large antigen load would tend to drive the response toward a Th2-type response predominance (Aaby, 1995; Bretscher et al., 1992; Hernandez-Pando and Rook, 1994). The measles vaccine, when used at the standard dose, reduced mortality by considerably more than can be accounted for by the incidence of measles in the unvaccinated population. It has been reported that diphtheria, tetanus, and pertussis (DPT) vaccines (Th2-inducing) do not show this nonspecific protective effect (Aaby et al., 1995). However, when a high-titer measles vaccine was used, the mortality increased, although protection from measles itself was maintained (Aaby, 1995; Aaby et al., 1995). There is evidence that this increase in mortality was accompanied by a switch toward a Th2-type response, and dose-related increases in the induction of a Th2-type component are well established for several other immunogens (Bretscher et al., 1992; Hernandez-Pando and Rook, 1994).

Third, the vaccinations were given after deployment of the troops in the war zone, or just before they traveled there, at a time when stress levels would have been high. Immunization in the presence of raised levels of glucocorticoids (i.e., cortisol) drives the cytokine expression response by stimulated lymphocytes toward a Th2-type predominance (Bernton et al., 1995; Brinkmann and Kristofic, 1995; Zwilling, 1992). Several steroid hormones modulate T-cell responses. The nervous, endocrine, and immune systems respond to internal and external challenges and communicate and regulate each other by means of shared or system-unique hormones, growth factors, neurotransmitters, and neuromodulators. For instance, similar alterations in central catecholamine neurotransmitter levels are associated with immune activity and stressor exposure—alterations that are more pronounced in aged as opposed to younger animals (Shanks et al., 1994). For example, a decreased norepinephrine turnover in the hypothalami and brainstem of rats occurs at the peak of the immune response to sheep red blood cells (Besedovsky et al., 1983; Vasina et al., 1975), and increased serotonin metabolism is associated with depressed Arthus reaction and plaque-forming cell response in rats stressed either by overcrowding lasting two weeks or more or by repeated immobilization for four days (Boranic, 1990; Boranic et al., 1982). The long-term effects of these acute changes are evidenced by chronic variable stress that facilitates tumor growth (Basso et al., 1992) and is associated with immune dysregulation in multiple sclerosis (Foley et al., 1992). The hypothalamic-pituitary-adrenal axis plays a pivotal role in stress-mediated changes, and stimulation of corticotropin-releasing factor in the CNS (De Souza, 1993; Irwin, 1993) has been shown to rapidly suppress a variety of immune responses, an effect that can be blocked by infusion into the brain of alpha-melanocyte-stimulating hormone, a tridecapeptide derived from pro-opiomelanocortin (Weiss et al., 1994).

Besides external stimuli, intrinsic imbalances in neurotransmitter levels affect the immune system either directly by acting on immunocompetent cells or indirectly via induction of hormonal secretions. For instance, depression is associated with neurotransmitter imbalances and with decreased natural killer cell cytotoxic activity (Hebert and Cohen, 1993; Irwin, Caldwell, et al., 1990; Irwin, Patterson, et al., 1990; Schleifer et al., 1989). Moreover, several studies have documented the existence of striking physiologic, neuroendocrine, metabolic, and pharmacologic differences between depressed and normal subjects and between depressed and severely ill subjects (Lechin, van der Dijs, Acosta, et al., 1983; Lechin, van der Dijs, Gomez, et al., 1983). Dehydroepiandrosterone (DHEA) or unknown metabolites of DHEA, tend to promote a Th1-type response pattern.

Thus, DHEA can restore immune functions in aged mice through correction of dysregulated cytokine release (Daynes et al., 1993; Garg and Bondade, 1993). DHEA has been tested for similar properties in aged humans (Morales et al., 1994) and found to enhance production of Th1-type cytokines, such as interleukin(IL)-2 and interferon(IFN)-gamma (Daynes and Araneo, 1989; Daynes et al., 1990, 1991, 1995). DHEA also enhances IL-2 secretion from human peripheral blood T cells (Suzuki et al., 1991). These effects of DHEA are the reverse of the effects of glucocorticoids such as cortisol, which enhance Th2-type response activity and synergize with Th2-type cytokines (Fischer and Konig, 1991; Guida et al., 1994; Padgett et al., 1995; Wu et al., 1991). If proliferation of naive T lymphocytes is driven in the presence of a nonspecific stimulus (Brinkmann and Kristofic, 1995) or by an antigen (as follows vaccination), T lymphocytes with a Th2-type cytokine profile will develop. This has been rather clearly shown with spleen cells from laboratory rodents that have few memory cells under normal circumstances (Zwilling, 1992). Overall, cortisol favors the development of a Th2-type cytokine profile form naive cells (Brinkmann and Kristofic, 1995). This point must not be confused with the fact that the cytokine-secreting activity of established Th2-type cells is readily inhibited by cortisol. Thus, the use of cortisol analogs for conventional treatments of Th2-mediated diseases, such as eczema, asthma, and hay fever may work via anti-inflammatory effects, and by reducing cytokine production by Th2-type cells (Corrigan et al., 1995), and yet at the same time the use of cortisol will encourage perpetuation of the underlying problem by driving newly recruited T cells toward a Th2-type response.

Psychological and physical stress activate the hypothalamic-pituitary-adrenal axis and thereby lead to a variety of changes including increased production of cortisol. In this respect, excessive exercise and deprivation of food and sleep result in a falling ratio of DHEA to cortisol. The latter falling ratio correlates directly with a fall in delayed hypersensitivity (DTH) responsiveness (a Th1-type response marker), and there is a simultaneous rise in serum IgE levels. IgE is wholly dependent upon Th2-type cytokine production (Bernton et al., 1995). This is to be expected in the light of known effects of DHEA and cortisol outlined previously. A further example of the effect of stress on Th1- to Th2-type switching is the increase in antibody to Epstein-Barr virus in students reacting in a stressed manner to their exams. This virus is usually controlled by a Th1-type response and cytotoxic T cells. Loss of control results in virus replication and increased antibody production (Glaser et al., 1993). Similarly, peripheral blood leukocytes from medical students during exam periods showed lower mRNA for IFN-gamma, a Th1-type cytokine (Glaser et al., 1993). Similar points can be demonstrated in a more controlled manner in animals. Stress secondary to crowding or restraint can increase mycobacterial growth in tuberculosis mice (Brown et al., 1993; Tobach et al., 1956). This is a model that is acutely sensitive to the presence of even a small Th2 component (Rook and Hernandez-Pando, 1996; Rook and Stanford, 1996). In tuberculosis, there is a systemic shift to a Th2-type response predominance (Rook and Hernandez-Pando, 1996; Rook and Stanford, 1996), and an unusual pattern of metabolites of adrenal steroids is excreted in the urine (Rook and Stanford, 1996). Treatment of the disease restores the Th1-type predominance and corrects the pattern of steroid metabolites, so that metabolites of cortisone increase relative to metabolites of cortisol (Rook and Hernandez-Pando, 1996; Rook and Stanford, 1996). There is considerable evidence that depression can be associated with excessive cortisol-mediated effects in the brain (Raven et al., 1995, 1996), and stress can lead to depression. Thus, depression (as seen in CFS and Gulf War syndrome) tends to associate with Th2-mediated disorders, such as asthma and eczema, and some endocrine changes are common to Th2 disorders and to depression (Holsboer et al., 1984; Rupprecht et al., 1996). Treatment of depression with the drug metyrapone causes the same change in steroid metabolites (e.g., increase in metabolites of cortisone relative to metabolites of cortisol) as those described previously after treatment of tuberculosis (Holsboer et al., 1984; Raven et al., 1996).

Fourth, Gulf War troops were also exposed to carbamate and organophosphorus insecticides, and these inhibit IL-2-driven phenomena essential for normal Th1-type function (Casale et al., 1993). The importance of this component is uncertain. However, it has been rumored that the insecticides were often obtained from local sources in the Gulf so purity was not known, and even more toxic contaminants may have been present.

Thus, multiple vaccinations administered under these circumstances may have caused a long-lasting systemic cytokine imbalance. The same effect would occur sporadically in the general population, secondary to vaccinations or other Th2-type response-inducing environmental stimuli and infections, and could account for the widespread incidence of CFS. It should be stressed at this point that not all vaccines and infectious agents induce a preponderance of the Th2-type response. For instance, measles infection reduced the incidence of atopy and of allergic reactions to house dust mites (Shaheen et al., 1996). Similarly, Japanese children that are tuberculin skin-test positive are less likely to be atopic than are tuberculin-negative children, and their ratio of circulating Th1/Th2 cytokines is higher. Moreover, after repeated injection of Bacillus Camelet-Guerin (BCG), those in whom tuberculin conversion occurs have an increased probability of losing their atopic symptoms.

Chapter 8

Immunotherapy
of Chronic Fatigue Syndrome:
Th1/Th2 Balance Modulation

Based on the postulates of viral and autoimmune etiologies of CFS, several interventions have been designed and tested by different research groups around the world, including the United States, Sweden, United Kingdom, Italy, and Japan. Patients with CFS who show evidence of activation of the immune system have poor immune cell function and a predominance of what is called a T-helper (Th)2-type cytokine response when their lymphocytes are activated. A Th2-type response, which is characterized by production of cytokines such as interleukin (IL)-4, -5, and -10, favors the function of B lymphocytes, the cellular factories of immunoglobulins. A predominance of a Th2-type response is therefore consistent with pathologies, such as autoimmunity and atopy, which are based on inappropriate production of immunoglobulins. Many of the CFS therapies discussed decrease the Th2-type predominance seen at baseline in CFS patients, thereby allowing a greater predominance of a Th1-type response, which favors the function of macrophages and natural killer cells. The function of the latter cells, which have the natural ability of directly destroying invading microbes and cancer cells, is defective in untreated CFS patients. Typical Th1-type cytokines include IL-2 and interferon-gamma, and some of the therapies induce their production. The interventions discussed in this chapter cover a wide spectrum of therapeutic tools ranging from lymph node cell-based immunotherapy, herbal products, and small molecules to vaccines. Despite the controversies on the etiology of CFS, immunotherapy research is useful and necessary.

Although vaccines, stressful stimuli, and some pathogens have been shown to lead to long-term, nonspecific shifts in cytokine balance (Aaby, 1995; Aaby et al., 1995; Mu and Sewell, 1993), the factors that could lead to a Th2 shift in CFS patients are unknown. Nevertheless, several therapeutic regimens that induce a systemic Th1 bias, some based on the use of certain vaccines, are being tested with preliminary success in subpopulations of CFS patients with documented baseline immune abnormalities. Moreover, whether directly or indirectly, viruses may play a role in the etiology or the perpetuation of symptoms of CFS. Some authors have put forth the notion that reactivation of latent viruses, if not etiological, may serve as a perpetuation factor for CFS symptomatology and may account for the remission-exacerbation cycling nature of the disease. On the other hand, viral reactivation may be an epiphenomenon and not necessarily related to symptomatology. Although mainly focused on therapeutic interventions, this chapter addresses therapies based on the hypotheses discussed above and others on how local and/or systemic effects of acute or reactivated viral activity may underlie CFS.

The first half of the twentieth century witnessed the first successful approach to control the spread of several viral infections: the development and worldwide use of vaccines. The concept of vaccination was originally developed by Jenner in eighteenth-century England based on the observation that milkmaids exposed to cows with cowpox were protected from smallpox. In this case, a subclinical infection with one virus was protective of an infection with a related one. The latter concept was also extended to the treatment of various infectious diseases by giving to the patient even unrelated but more innocuous infectious diseases. Although in many cases the treatment was worse than the disease, the therapeutic approach was somehow useful with particular combinations of infectious agents.

Outstanding triumphs from worldwide vaccination programs have been the eradication of smallpox and predictably soon of poliomyelitis (Marwick, 2000). After smallpox was eliminated as an infectious disease in Great Britain in 1962, two outbreaks occurred, one in 1973 and one in 1978, when smallpox virus under study in laboratories infected susceptible individuals. In both incidents, deaths resulted (Marwick, 2000). With the eradication of poliomyelitis throughout the world soon to be accomplished, steps are being taken to prevent polioviruses that remain in laboratories from escaping into the community and causing disease. These examples stress the need for universal availability of vaccines to effectively eradicate the disease they cause. Unfortunately, we do not have vaccines against all viruses and even in the cases for which we do, the vaccine is not universally available. The dramatic success in immunizing children against childhood diseases stands in stark contrast to the much lower percentages of adults who are adequately immunized against common adult diseases. In the case of the flu vaccine, the influenza virus keeps changing and the vaccine must be updated every year, and it is therefore not fully protective against all viral strains.

One alternative to vaccines has been the use of injections of immunoglobulins, the natural bullets that the body produces to kill foreign invaders. Not too long ago, physicians advocated the use of immunoglobulin injections as a way to boost the body's immune defenses and heighten resistance against microbes. The latter reasoning was perhaps again reflective of the old wisdom of using one infection to protect against another with the added refinement of using the natural mediators of the body's attack machinery against infections instead of the infectious agent itself. The following therapeutic interventions are based on the use of vaccines and the modulation of the body's defenses using certain microbes.

LYMPH NODE CELL-BASED IMMUNOTHERAPY

Lymph nodes are an attractive source of cells for immune modulation. They contain all the critical elements to develop an immune response, including antigen-presenting cells (A.C.). Also, the yield of immunologically active cells can be orders of magnitude greater than that from the peripheral blood. Lymph nodes often sequester virus and virus-specific cytotoxic T lymphocytes in an efficient system designed to eliminate or control viral infection. The expression of specific adhesion molecules and the locomotor capability of lymph node lymphocytes, and thus the ability to traffic, may also be superior to that of the peripheral blood mononuclear cells (Tedla et al., 1999).

Nancy Klimas, Mary Ann Fletcher, and Roberto Patarca, at the University of Miami, completed a safety and feasibility study using lymph node extraction, ex vivo cell culture, followed by autologous cell reinfusion as a treatment strategy to favor a Th2- to Th1-type cytokine expression shift in selected CFS patients (Klimas and Fletcher, 1999; Klimas et al., 2000; Patarca et al., 2000). Lymph nodes were obtained from patients who met the current case definition for CFS and the following inclusion criteria: a history of acute onset; a Karnofsky score less than 80; evidence of immune dysfunction in three or more of the following: greater than one standard deviation above controls for elevated soluble TNF receptor type I (sTNF-RI) levels in serum, elevated sTNF-RI production in phytohemmaglutinin (PHA)-stimulated blood culture, or elevated IL-5 production in PHA-stimulated blood culture; lymphocyte activation (CD2+CD26+ cells > 50 percent); or low NK cell cytotoxic activity (< 20 percent). The lymph node cells were cultured for ten to twelve days with anti-CD3 and IL-2. These cells were then reinfused into the donor who was monitored for safety and possible clinical benefit. There were no adverse events noted in this Phase 1 clinical trial. Of thirteen subjects, two had palpable lymph nodes that proved fiber optic with no viable cells. Of the remaining eleven subjects, all successfully underwent expansion and reinfusion. In some of the patients, there was an elevation in the expression of IL-2 receptor on CD4 T cells in the weeks following the reinfusion. There was a significant decrease in IL-5 production by PHA-stimulated blood cultures observed at one week, which persisted for several weeks postinfusion. Levels of PHA-induced IFN-gamma production did not change. There was a trend toward an increase in the ratio of IFN-gamma/IL-5 starting at week one and persisting at least twelve weeks postinfusion. Of the eleven subjects in the trial who had cells reinfused, nine had significant cognitive improvement. There was a trend toward significant change in speed of visual scanning (Trailmaking Test A). There was a significant increase in the patients' ability to mentally track and rapidly shift cognitive set, as measured in Trailmaking Test B. Other measures of severity of illness also trended toward improvement. There was a significant increase in Karnofsky and Symptom Impact Profile scores, and a significant association between clinical improvement and IFN-gamma/IL-5 (Th1/Th2) ratio increase. Six patients showed both clinical improvement and Th1/Th2 ratios; four showed neither clinical improvement nor increased Th1/Th2 ratios; and only one patient had a significant clinical improvement and no change in the Th1/Th2 ratio. The lack of adverse effects from this experimental approach to immunomodulation in CFS and the favorable clinical and immunologic results observed in the small number of patients studied suggest that further clinical trials are warranted.

These studies on CFS patients were preceded by studies of adoptive CD8+ T-cell immunotherapy of AIDS patients with Kaposi's sarcoma (Klimas, 1992; Klimas et al., 1993; Klimas, Patarca, Maher, et al., 1994; Klimas, Patarca, Walling, et al., 1994; Patarca, Klimas, et al., 1994; Patarca, Klimas, Walling, et al., 1995). The research group used a device developed to selectively capture CD8+ T cells for ex vivo culture and instituted basic science and clinical evaluations of the consequences of the infusion, with rIL-2, of autologous, activated, and polyclonally expanded CD8+ T cells in AIDS patients with Kaposi's sarcoma and oral hairy leukoplakia. Phase I and II trials showed safety and suggested efficacy in the treatment of the latter AIDS-associated conditions. The intervention affected the patterns of cytokine expression of CD8+ T lymphocytes and favored a restoration of a strong type 1 response (Patarca, Klimas, Walling, et al., 1995).

MYCOBACTERIUM VACCAE

As described in internationally published patent number WO-09826790 by Rook, Stanford, and Zumla, preparations of killed *Mycobacterium vaccae* are able to effect a nonspecific systemic Th1-type response bias, in particular by down-regulation of Th2-type activity without concomitant up-regulation of Th1-type activity. The latter feature is similar to the effect on the Th1/Th2 type proportions of the lymph node cell-based immunotherapy previously described.

In experimental animals, a nonspecific systemic bias away from Th2-type activity on administration of *M. vaccae* can be seen as a reduction in the titer of an IL-4 (Th2)-dependent antibody response to ovalbumin (an allergen unrelated to *M. vaccae* itself), in mice pre-immunized so as to establish a Th2-type response. A single injection of *M. vaccae* is able to cause this effect and further injections can enhance it. The effect is nonspecific because it does not require the presence of any component of ovalbumin in the injected preparation.

Briefly, BALB/c mice six to eight weeks old were immunized with 50 μg ovalbumin emulsified in oil (incomplete Freund's adjuvant) on days 0 and 24. This is known to evoke a strong Th2-type pattern of response, accompanied by IgE production, and priming for release of two Th2-type cytokines, IL-4 and IL-5. Animals then received saline or 10^7 autoclaved *M. vaccae* on days 53 and 81 by subcutaneous injection. Injections of *M. vaccae* reduced the rise in IgE levels caused by immunization with ovalbumin. The reduction caused by treatment with *M. vaccae* was significant at all time points tested. Similarly, spleen cells from the immunized animals failed to release IL-5 in vitro in response to ovalbumin if the donor animals had been treated with *M. vaccae,* although spleen cells from immunized animals treated with saline released large quantities of IL-5 in response to ovalbumin. The latter data shows that *M. vaccae* will reduce a Th2-type pattern of response, even when given after immunization with a potent allergen, and without epitopes of the Th2-inducing molecule. There is therefore a nonspecific systemic down-regulation of the Th2-type pattern of response, not dependent upon a direct adjuvant effect on the allergen itself.

In cancer patients, the effect of *M. vaccae* injection has been demonstrated by the appearance in the peripheral blood of lymphocytes that spontaneously secrete IL-2 (a characteristic Th1 cytokine) and decrease in T cells that secrete IL-4 (a characteristic Th2 cytokine) after stimulation with phorbol myristate acetate and calcium ionophore. The percentage of lymphocytes showing this activated Th1-type phenotype increases progressively after each successive injection of *M. vaccae,* reaching a plateau in many individuals after three to five injections of 10^9 organisms (days 0, 15, 30, and then monthly).

The *M. vaccae* used for these therapies is grown on a solid medium including modified Sauton's medium solidified with 1.3 percent agar. The medium is inoculated with the microorganisms and incubated aerobically for ten days at 32°C to enable growth of the microorganism to take place. The microorganisms are then harvested and weighed and suspended in diluent to give 100 mg of microorganisms/mL of diluent. The suspension is then further diluted with buffered saline to give a suspension containing 10 mg wet weight (about 10^{10} cells) of microorganisms/mL of diluent and dispensed into 5 mL multidose vials. The vials containing the live microorganisms are then autoclaved (115 to 125°C) for ten minutes at 69 kPa to kill the microorganisms. The therapeutic agent thus produced is stored at 4°C before use. Then 0.1 mL of the suspension, containing 1 mg wet weight (about 10^9 cells) of *M. vaccae,* is shaken vigorously immediately before being administered by intradermal injection over the left deltoid muscle.

In the same patent publication, Rook, Stamford, and Zumla describe their experience with CFS patients treated with *M. vaccae*. For instance, a CFS patient reported improvement after two injections of a *M. vaccae* preparation. A second one reported that since she had been receiving a *M. vaccae* preparation at two-month intervals, her CFS symptoms and food allergy had improved considerably and she continues to feel very well as long as she continues with her regular injections.

STAPHYLOCOCCAL VACCINE

In international published patent number WO-09829133 by Goteborg University Science Invest AB, Carl-Gergard Gottfries and Bjoern Regland describe the use of staphylococcal vaccine to favor a Th1-type predominance. These authors also found that variables such as smoking and nickel sensitivity adversely affect the outcome of this form of therapy (Andersson et al., 1998). The treatment is preferably conducted as a series of administrations with increasing doses during a specific period. Preferably, the vaccine is administered in eight to ten increasing doses during four to twelve weeks, preferably for eight to ten weeks. The reason for the increasing doses is that during the first week or weeks, the patient will probably suffer from side effects, and it is therefore advantageous to start with a low dose. The side effects will diminish over time. The first series of administrations is followed by repeated administrations given approximately once a week for five to fifteen weeks, preferably for ten weeks. To prevent recurrence, the repeated administrations are then followed by a maintenance treatment with administrations approximately once a month, which preferably are continued for several years, such as one to ten years, preferably for approximately five years. The doses in the repeated administrations of the maintenance treatment are preferably constant and relatively high. Vitamin B_{12} and/or folacin is preferably administered simultaneously or in parallel with the staphylococcal preparation.

If the known staphylococcal vaccine Staphypan Berna from the Serum and Vaccine Institute, Bern, Switzerland, is used, a typical treatment schedule may be as follows: eight to ten administrations are made during a period of four to twelve weeks, preferably eight to ten weeks, wherein the dose of the staphylococcal preparation is gradually increased from 0.1 to 1 mL of the pure vaccine. The increase depends on the response from the patient. It may be, for example, 0.1, 0.2, 0.3, 0.4, 0.5, 0.6, 0.7, 0.8, 0.9, and 1.0 mL, respectively. If the patient shows a strong local reaction, it is possible to repeat a dose before increasing it. The dose of staphylococcal preparation in the repeated administration and in maintenance treatment is 1 mL.

As described in the published patent, after a pilot study comprising eight patients was made, a double-blind placebo-controlled study was performed, comprising a group of twenty-four female adult patients fulfilling both the criteria for fibromyalgia and for chronic fatigue syndrome. Seven of the thirteen patients who received the staphylococcal preparation were assessed as being minimally improved, three as being much improved, and the remaining three were unchanged. In the placebo group, three patients were minimally improved, and the remaining eight were unchanged. The improvement in the group with active treatment was statistically significant ($p < 0.05$) compared to the improvement in the placebo group. Following the controlled study, twenty-four patients chose to continue with the treatment and twenty of these have been treated for between one and two years. Nineteen of these twenty patients were on the sick list or received sickness pension prior to the start of treatment, and one patient was employed part-time. At a one-year follow-up after the completed study, nine of the twenty patients were in full- or part-time paid employment; one patient was taking part in a work experience program; and one was at the middle of a two-year training to become a nurse. The treatment strategy used in this study is a series of administrations of staphylococcal preparations given approximately once a week during a period of some months, for example, three months and thereafter long-term treatment with monthly administrations. Further studies are being conducted by this Swedish group.

SIZOFIRAN

Sizofiran, an immunostimulant extracted from suehirotake mushroom *(Schizophyllum commune)* cultured fluid, is under development by Fidia Farmaceutici Italiani Deriviate Industriali e Affini for the potential treatment of cancer and hepatitis B. Sizofiran is licensed by Kaken Pharmaceutical Co., Ltd., Japan. Trials were under way for the treatment of gastric and lung tumor; Phase III trials are under way for the treatment of hepatitis B; and the compound is in Phase II trials for chronic fatigue syndrome. By August 1999, Kaken was preparing its NDA filing for hepatitis B, but no information is available regarding its status today.

Significant sizofiran-induced rises in IFN-gamma and IL-2 in culture medium of phytohemagglutinin (PHA) or concanavalin A-stimulated peripheral blood mononuclear cells have been observed. Further reports on sizofiran should become available in the near future.

PANAX GINSENG

In one study, an extract of the herb *Panax ginseng* was evaluated for its capacity to stimulate cellular immune function by peripheral blood mononuclear cells (PBMC) from normal individuals and patients with chronic fatigue syndrome. PBMC isolated on a Ficoll-Hypaque density gradient were tested in the presence or absence of varying concentrations of the extract for natural killer (NK) cell cytotoxic activity directed against K562 cell targets and for antibody-dependent cellular cytotoxicity (ADCC) directed against human herpesvirus 6-infected H9 cells. Ginseng, at concentrations greater or equal to 10 µg/kg, significantly enhanced NK cell function in both groups. Similarly, the addition of the herb significantly increased ADCC of PBMC from the subject groups. Thus, an extract of *Panax ginseng* enhances cellular immune function of PBMC from normal individuals as well as from patients with depressed cellular immunity and CFS (See et al., 1997). In line with the latter observations, ginseng treatment was found in another study to lead to activation of neutrophils and modulation of the immunoglobulin G response to *Pseudomonas aeruginosa,* thereby enhancing the bacterial clearance and reducing the formation of immune complexes, effects which resulted in a milder lung pathology in chronic *Pseudomonas aeruginosa* lung infection in cystic fibrosis patients. The therapeutic effects of ginseng may be related to activation of a Th1-type of cellular immunity and down-regulation of humoral immunity (Song et al., 1998).

Although ginseng is generally well tolerated, it has been implicated as a cause of decreased response to warfarin and may interfere with either digoxin pharmacodynamically or with digoxin monitoring (Cupp, 1999; McRae, 1996; Miller, 1998). Nevertheless, some authors claim no relationship between cardiac glycosides and glycosides in ginseng and attribute the effect on digoxin on contaminants (Awang, 1996; Wong, 1999). In addition, ginseng may cause headache, tremulousness, and manic episodes in patients treated with phenelzine sulfate. Ginseng should also not be used with estrogens or corticosteroids because of possible additive effects. Ginseng may affect blood glucose levels and should not be used in patients with diabetes mellitus (Miller, 1998).

JUZEN-TAIHO-TO

A group of Japanese herbal medicines called Hozai have been used to improve the physical condition of the elderly. One representative Hozai, Juzen-Taiho-To, was shown to modulate antigen-specific T-cell responses toward more balanced Th1/Th2-type responses in old BALB/c mice, which have a preferential Th-2 type cytokine response pattern (Lijima et al., 1999). Such effects may help prevent the development of diseases associated with immunodysregulation, including chronic fatigue syndrome.

Chapter 9

Concluding Remarks

The data summarized herein indicate that CFS is associated with immune abnormalities that can potentially account for physio- and psychopathological symptomatology. Assessment of immune status reveals a heterogeneity among CFS patients that allows their categorization, thus systematizing the study of the interactions among immune, psychological, and physiological parameters in this disorder. The study of immune status at different levels also provides an integrated view of this complex syndrome and is opening doors for deciphering its cause and for developing rational treatment protocols. Future research should further elucidate the cellular basis for immune dysfunction in CFS and its implications. Other compartments such as the CNS have to be assessed using similar techniques to those used with peripheral blood. Nonetheless, the studies in peripheral blood have been providing insight into the physio- and psychopathologies of CFS.

Immunotherapy of CFS holds promise and is an area of intense research that is being fed by a plethora of sources from herbal medicine, vaccines, and cell therapy to small molecules. Although the mechanisms whereby alterations in the immune system lead to changes in cognitive and functional status remain to be elucidated, the results of the different trials reinforce the need to integrate immunological, endocrinological, and psychological approaches to the understanding of the different manifestations of CFS. Some of the clinical trials also emphasize the importance of appropriately categorizing patients for interventions and outcome assessments. The experience garnered with CFS appears applicable to related conditions such as fibromyalgia, Gulf War syndrome, sick building syndrome, and multiple chemical sensitivity. The etiology of CFS remains elusive, but therapeutic intervention studies are opening the doors to control this ailment.

References

Aaby P. (1995). Assumptions and contradictions in measles and measles immunization research: Is measles good for something? *Social Sciences Medicine* 41(5):673-686.

Aaby P, Samb B, Simondon F, Seck AM, Knudsen K, Whittle H. (1995). Non-specific beneficial effect of measles immunization: Analysis of mortality studies from developing countries. *British Medical Journal* 311(7003):481-485.

Ablashi DV, Eastman HB, Owen CB, Roman MM, Friedman J, Zabriskie JB, Peterson DL, Pearson GR, Whitman JE. (2000). Frequent HHV-6 reactivation in multiple sclerosis (MS) and chronic fatigue syndrome (CFS) patients. *Journal of Clinical Virology* 16(3):179-191.

Ablashi DV, Handy M, Bernbaum J, Chatlynne LG, Lapps W, Kramarsky B, Berneman ZN, Komaroff AL, Whitman JE. (1998). Propagation and characterization of human herpes virus-7 (HHV-7) isolates in a continuous T-lymphoblastoid cell line (SUPT1). *Journal of Virological Methods* 73(2):123-140.

Ablashi DV, Kramarsky B, Bernbaum J, Whitman JE, Pearson GR. (1995). Viruses and chronic fatigue syndrome: Current status. *Journal of Chronic Fatigue Syndrome* 1:3-22.

Alheim K, McDowell TL, Symons JA, Duff GW, Bartfai T. (1996). An AP-1 site is involved in the NGF induction of IL-1 alpha in PC12 cells. *Neurochemistry International* 29:487.

Allain TJ, Bearn JA, Coskeran P, Jones J, Checkley A, Butler J, Wessely S, Miell JP. (1997). Changes in growth hormone, insulin, insulin like growth factors (IGFs), and IGF-binding protein-1 in chronic fatigue syndrome. *Biological Psychiatry* 41(5):567-573.

Alpert S, Kloide J, Takada S, Engleman EG. (1987). T-cell regulatory disturbances in the rheumatic diseases. *Rheumatic Diseases Clinics of North America* 13(3): 431-435.

Altman C, Larratt K, Golubjatnikov R. (1988). Immunologic markers in the chronic fatigue syndrome. *Clinical Research* 36:845A.

Alviggi L, Johnson C, Hoskins PJ, Tee DE, Pyke DA, Leslie RD, Vergani D. (1984). Pathogenesis of insulin-dependent diabetes: A role for activated T lymphocytes. *Lancet* 2:4-6.

Andersson M, Bagby JR, Dyrehag LE, Gottfries CG. (1998). Effects of staphylococcal toxoid vaccine on pain and fatigue in patients with fibromyalgia/chronic fatigue syndrome. *European Journal of Pain* 2:133-142.

Andondonskaja-Renz B, Zeitler H. (1984). Pteridines in plasma and in cells of peripheral blood tumor patients. In *Biochemical and Clinical Aspects of Pteridines*, Pfeiderer W, Wachter H, Curtius HC (Eds.). Berlin-New York, Walter de Gruyter, pp. 295-311.

Anisman H, Baines MG, Berczi I, Bernstein CN, Blennerhassett MG, Gorczynski RM, Greenberg AH, Kisil FT, Mathison RD, Nagy E, Nance DM, Perdue MH, Pomerantz DK, Sabbadini ER, Stanisz A, Warrington RJ. (1996). Neuroimmune mechanisms in health and disease: 2. Disease. *Canadian Medical Association Journal* 155(8):1075-1082.

Aoki T, Usada Y, Miyakoshi H. (1985). A novel immunodeficiency: Low NK syndrome (LNKS). *Japanese Journal of Medicine* 3212:14-17.

Aoki T, Usuda Y, Miyakoshi H, Tamura K, Herberman RB. (1987). Low natural syndrome: Clinical and immunologic features. *Natural Immunity and Cell Growth Regulation* 6(3):116-128.

Archard LC, Bowles NE, Behan PO, Bell EJ, Doyle D. (1988). Post viral fatigue syndrome: Persistence of enterovirus RNA in muscle and elevated creatinine kinase. *Journal of the Royal Society of Medicine* 81:326-329.

Arnason BGW. (1991). Nervous system-immune system communication. *Review of Infectious Diseases* 13(1):S134-S137.

Asim M, Turney JH. (1997).The female patient with faints and fatigue: Don't forget Sjogren's syndrome. *Nephrology, Dialysis, Transplantation* 12(7):1516-1517.

Atkinson MA, Bowman MA, Campbell L, Darrow BL, Kaufman DL, Maclaren NK. (1994). Cellular immunity to a determinant common in glutamate decarboxylase and coxsackievirus in insulin-dependent diabetes. *Journal of Clinical Investigation* 94(5):2125-2129.

Awang DVC. (1996). Siberian ginseng toxicity may be case of mistaken identity. *Canadian Medical Association Journal* 155:1237.

Ayres JG, Flint N, Smith EG, Tunnicliffe WS, Fletcher TJ, Hammond K, Ward D, Marmion BP. (1998). Post-infection fatigue syndrome following Q fever. *Quarterly Journal of Medicine* 91(2):105-123.

Bagasra O, Fitzharis JW, Bagasra TT. (1988). Neopterin: An early marker of development of pre-AIDS conditions in HIV-seropositive individuals. *Clinical Immunology Newsletter* 9:197-199.

Baier-Bitterlich G, Fuchs D, Murr C, Reibnegger G, Werner Felmayer G, Sgonc R, Böck G, Dierich MP, Wachter H. (1995). Effect of neopterin and 7.8-dihydro-neopterin on tumor necrosis factor-alpha induced programmed cell death. *FEBS Letters* 364:234-238.

Banki K, Maceda J, Hurley E, Ablonczy E, Mattson DH, Szegedy L, Hung C, Perl A. (1992). Human T-cell lymphotropic virus (HTLV)-related endogenous sequence, HRES-1, encodes a 28-kDa protein: A possible autoantigen for HTLV-I gag reactive autoantibodies. *Proceedings of the National Academy of Sciences USA* 89(5):1939-1943.

Baraniuk JN, Clauw DJ, Gaumond E. (1998). Rhinitis symptoms in chronic fatigue syndrome. *Annals of Allergy, Asthma, and Immunology* 81(4):359-365.

Baraniuk JN, Clauw DJ, MacDowell-Carneiro AL, Bellanti J, Pandiri P, Foong S, Ali M. (1998). IgE concentrations in chronic fatigue syndrome. *Journal of Chronic Fatigue Syndrome* 4(1):13-22.

Barendregt PJ, Visser MR, Smets EM, Tulen JH, van den Meiracker AH, Boomsma F, Markusse HM. (1998). Fatigue in primary Sjogren's syndrome. *Annals of Rheumatic Diseases* 57(5):291-295.

Barker E, Fujimura SF, Fadem MB, Landay AL, Levy JA. (1994). Immunologic abnormalities associated with chronic fatigue syndrome. *Clinical Infectious Diseases* 18(Suppl. 1):S136-S141.

Baschetti R. (1996). High androgen levels in chronic fatigue patients. *Journal of Clinical Endocrinology and Metabolism* 81(7):2752-2753.

Baschetti R. (1997). Similarity of symptoms in chronic fatigue syndrome and Addison's disease. *European Journal of Clinical Investigation* 27(12):1061-1062.

Baschetti R. (1999a). Cortisol deficiency may account for elevated apoptotic cell population in patients with chronic fatigue syndrome. *Journal of Internal Medicine* 245(4):409-410.

Baschetti R. (1999b). Investigations of hydrocortisone and fludrocortisone in the treatment of chronic fatigue syndrome. *Journal of Endocrinology and Metabolism* 84(6):2263-2264.

Baschetti R. (1999c). Low-dose hydrocortisone for chronic fatigue syndrome. *Journal of the American Medical Association* 281(20):1887.

Baschetti R. (1999d). Overlap of chronic fatigue syndrome with primary adrenocortical insufficiency. *Hormone and Metabolism Research* 31(7):439.

Basso AM, Depiante-Depaoli M, Molina VA. (1992). Chronic variable stress facilitates tumoral growth: Reversal by imipramine administration. *Life Sciences* 50(23):1789-1796.

Bates DW, Buchwald D, Lee J, Kith P, Doolittle T, Rutherford C, Churchill WH, Schur PH, Werner M, Wybenga D, et al. (1995). Clinical laboratory test findings in patients with chronic fatigue syndrome. *Archives of Internal Medicine* 155(1):97-103.

Behan PO, Behan WHM, Bell EJ. (1985). The postviral fatigue syndrome—An analysis of the findings in 50 cases. *Journal of Infectious Diseases* 10:211-222.

Bennett AL, Chao CC, Hu S, Buchwald D, Fagioli LR, Schur PH, Peterson PK, Komaroff AL. (1997). Elevation of bioactive transforming growth factor-beta in serum from patients with chronic fatigue syndrome. *Journal of Clinical Immunology* 17(2):160-166.

Bennett AL, Fagioli LR, Schur PH, Schacterle RS, Komaroff AL. (1996). Immunoglobulin subclass levels in chronic fatigue syndrome. *Journal of Clinical Immunology* 16(6):315-320.

Bennett AL, Mayes DM, Fagioli LR, Guerriero R, Komaroff AL. (1997). Somtomedin C (insulin-like growth factor I) levels in patients with chronic fatigue syndrome. *Journal of Psychiatric Research* 31(1):91-96.

Bennett BK, Hickie IB, Vollmer-Conna US, Quigley B, Brennan CM, Wakefield D, Douglas MP, Hansen GR, Tahmindjis AJ, Lloyd AR. (1998). The relationship between fatigue, psychological and immunological variables in acute infectious illness. *Australia and New Zealand Journal of Psychiatry* 32(2):180-186.

Berg D, Berg LH, Couvaras J, Harison H. (1999). Chronic fatigue syndrome and/or fibromyalgia as a variation of antiphospholipid antibody syndrome: An explanatory model and approach to laboratory diagnosis. *Blood Coagulation and Fibrinolysis* 10(7):435-438.

Berkenbosch F, Van Oers J, Del Rey A, Tilders F, Besedovsky H. (1987). Corticotropin-releasing factor-producing neurons in the RT activated by interleukin-1. *Science* 238:524-526.

Bernton EW, Beach J, Holaday JW, Smallridge RC, Fein HG. (1987). Release of multiple hormones by a direct action of interleukin-1 on pituitary cells. *Science* 238:519-521.

Bernton EW, Hoover D, Galloway R, Popp K. (1995). Adaptation to chronic stress in military trainees: Adrenal androgens, testosterone, glucocorticoids, IGF-1, and immune function. *Annals of the New York Academy of Sciences* 774:217-231.

Berwaerts J, Moorkens G, Abs R. (1998). Review of neuroendocrine disturbances in the chronic fatigue syndrome: Indications for a role of the growth hormone-IGF-1 axis in the pathogenesis. *Journal of Chronic Fatigue Syndrome* 4(4):81-92.

Besedovsky H, del Rey A, Sorkin E, Da Prada M, Burri R, Honegger C. (1983). The immune response evokes changes in brain noradrenergic neurons. *Science* 221(4610):564-566.

Besedovsky H, del Rey A, Sorkin E, Dinarello CA. (1986). Immunoregulatory feedback between interleukin-1 and glucocorticoid hormones. *Science* 233:652-654.

Best CL, Hill JA. (1995). Interleukin-1 alpha and beta modulation of luteinized human granulosa cell oestrogen and progesterone biosynthesis. *Human Reproduction* 10:3206.

Beutler B., Cerami A. (1988). Cachectin (tumor necrosis factor). A macrophage hormone governing cellular metabolism and inflammatory response. *Endocrinological Reviews* 9:57-66.

Black RB, Leong AS, Crowed PA. (1980). Lymphocyte subpopulations in human lymph nodes: A normal range. *Lymphology* 13:86-90.

Blick M, Bresser J, Lepe-Zuniga JL, Goodacre A, Luethke D, Holder WR, Duvic M. (1990). Identification of human immunodeficiency virus hybridizing sequences in the peripheral blood of a patient with systemic lupus erythematosus. *Journal of the American Academy of Dermatology* 23(4Pt1):641-645.

Blum-Degen D, Muller T, Kuhn W, Gerlach M, Przuntek H, Riederer P. (1995). Interleukin-1 beta and interleukin-6 are elevated in the cerebrospinal fluid of Alzheimer's and de novo Parkinson's disease patients. *Neurosciences Letters* 202:17.

Bode L, Fersyt R, Czech G. (1993). Borna disease virus infection and affective disorders in man. *Archives of Virology* 7:159-167.

Boranic M. (1990). The central nervous system and immunity. *Lijecnicki Vjesnik* 112(9-10):329-334.

Boranic M, Pericic D, Radacic M, Poljak-Blasi M, Sverko V, Miljenovic G. (1982). Immunological and neuroendocrine responses of rats to prolonged or repeated stress. *Biomedicine and Pharmacotherapy* 36(1):23-28.

Borish L, Schmaling K, DiClementi JD, Streib J, Negri J, Jones JF. (1998). Chronic fatigue syndrome: Identification of distinct subgroups on the basis of allergy and psychological variables. *Journal of Allergy and Clinical Immunology* 102(2):222-230.

Borok G. (1998). Chronic fatigue syndrome: An atopic state. *Journal of Chronic Fatigue Syndrome* 4(3):39-58.

Borysiewicz LK, Haworth SJ, Cohen J, Munin J, Rickinson A, Sissons JG. (1986). Epstein-Barr virus-specific immune defects in patients with persistent symptoms following infectious mononucleosis. *Quarterly Journal of Medicine* 58:111-121.

Bottero P. (2000). Role of Rickettsiae and Chlamydiae in the psychopathology of chronic fatigue syndrome (CFS) patients: A diagnostic and therapeutic report. *Journal of Chronic Fatigue Syndrome* 6(3/4):147-161.

Bounous G, Molson J. (1999). Competition for glutamine precursors between the immune system and the skeletal muscle: Pathogenesis of chronic fatigue syndrome. *Medical Hypotheses* 53(4):347-349.

Braun DK, Dominguez G, Pellett PE. (1997). Human herpesvirus 6. *Clinical Microbiology Reviews* 10(3):521-567.

Bretscher PA, Wei G, Menon JN, Bielefeldt-Ohmann H. (1992). Establishment of stable, cell-mediated immunity that makes "susceptible" mice resistant to *Leishmania major. Science* 257(5069):539-542.

Brinkmann V, Kristofic C. (1995). Regulation of corticosteroids of Th1 and Th2 cytokine production in human CD4+ effector T cells generated from CD45RO– and CD45RO+ subsets. *Journal of Immunology* 155(7):3322-3328.

Brown DH, Sheridan J, Pearl D, Zwilling BS. (1993). Regulation of mycobacterial growth by the hypothalamus-pituitary-adrenal axis: Differential responses of *Mycobacterium bovis*-BCG-resistant and -susceptible mice. *Infection and Immunity* 61(11):4793-4800.

Bruno RL, Creange SJ, Frick NM. (1998). Parallels between post-polio fatigue and chronic fatigue syndrome: A common pathophysiology? *American Journal of Medicine* 105(3A):66S-73S.

Bryan CF, Eastman J, Conner B, Baier KA, Durham JB. (1993). Clinical utility of a lymph node normal range obtained by flow cytometry. *Annals of the New York Academy of Sciences* 667:404-406.

Buchwald D, Ashley RL, Pearlman T, Kith P, Komaroff AL. (1996). Viral serologies in patients with chronic fatigue and chronic fatigue syndrome. *Journal of Medical Virology* 50(1):25-30.

Buchwald D, Cheney PR, Peterson DL, Henry B, Wormsley SB, Geiger A, Ablashi DV, Salahuddin SZ, Saxinger C, Biddle R, et al. (1992). A chronic illness characterized by fatigue, neurologic and immunologic disorders and active human herpesvirus 6 type infection. *Annals of Internal Medicine* 116(2):103-113.

Buchwald D, Komaroff AL. (1991). Review of laboratory findings for patients with chronic fatigue syndrome. *Review of Infectious Diseases* 13(1):S12-S18.

Buchwald D, Umali J, Stene M. (1996). Insulin-like growth factor-I (somatomedin C) levels in chronic fatigue syndrome and fibromyalgia. *Journal of Rheumatology* 23(4):739-742.

Buchwald D, Wener MH, Pearlman T, Kith P. (1997). Markers of inflammation and immune activation in chronic fatigue and chronic fatigue syndrome. *Journal of Rheumatology* 24(2):372-376.

Bujak DI, Weinstein A, Dornbush RL. (1996). Lyme disease. Clinical and neurocognitive features of the post Lyme syndrome. *Journal of Rheumatology* 23(8): 1392-1397.

Burroughs MH, Tsenova-Berkova L, Sokol K, Ossig J, Tuomanen E, Kaplan G. (1995). Effect of thalidomide on the inflammatory response in cerebrospinal fluid in experimental bacterial meningitis. *Microbial Pathogenesis* 19:245.

Calabrese JR, Kling MA, Gold PA. (1987). Alterations in immunocompetence during stress, bereavement, and depression: Focus on neuroendocrine regulation. *American Journal of Psychiatry* 144:1123-1134.

Caligiuri M, Murray C, Buchwald D, Levine H, Cheney P, Peterson D, Komaroff AL, Kitz J. (1987). Phenotypic and functional deficiency of natural killer cells in patients with chronic fatigue syndrome. *Journal of Immunology* 139(10):3306-3313.

Cannon JG, Angel JB, Abad LW, O'Grady J, Lundgren N, Fagioli L, Komaroff AL. (1998). Hormonal influences on stress-induced neutrophil mobilization in health and chronic fatigue syndrome. *Journal of Clinical Immunology* 18(4):291-298.

Cannon JG, Angel JB, Abad LW, Vannier E, Mileno MD, Fagioli L, Wolff SM, Komaroff AL. (1997). Interleukin-1 beta, interleukin-1 receptor antagonist, and soluble interleukin-1 receptor type II secretion in chronic fatigue syndrome. *Journal of Clinical Immunology* 17(3):253-261.

Cannon JG, Angel JB, Ball RW, Abad LW, Fagioli L, Komaroff AL. (1999). Acute phase responses and cytokine secretion in chronic fatigue syndrome. *Journal of Clinical Immunology* 19(6):414-421.

Canonica GW, Bagnasco M, Corte G, et al. (1982). Circulating T lymphocytes in Hashimoto's disease: Imbalance of subsets and presence of activated cells. *Clinical Immunology and Immunopathology* 23:616-625.

Cantor H, Boyse EA. (1977). Regulation of cellular and humoral immune responses by T-cell subclasses. *Cold Spring Harbor Symposia on Quantitative Biology* 41:23-32.

Casale GP, Vennerstrom JL, Bavari S, Wang TL. (1993). Inhibition of interleukin 2 driven proliferation of mouse CTLL2 cells, by selected carbamate and organophosphate insecticides and congeners of carbaryl. *Immunopharmacology and Immunotoxicology* 15(2-3):199-215.

Casali P, Notkins AL. (1989). CD5+ B lymphocytes, polyreactive antibodies and the human B cell repertoire. *Immunology Today* 10:364-368.

Caverzasio J, Rizzoli R, Dayer JM. (1987). Interleukin-1 decreases renal sodium reabsorption: Possible mechanisms of endotoxin-induced natriuresis. *American Journal of Physiology* 252:943-946.

Chai Z, Alheim K, Lundkvist J, Gatti S, Bartfai T. (1996). Subchronic glucocorticoid pretreatment reversily attenuates IL-1beta induced fever in rats; IL-6 mRNA is elevated while IL-1 alpha and IL-1 beta mRNAs are suppressed, in the CNS. *Cytokine* 8:227.

Chao CC, Gallagher M, Phair J, Peterson PK. (1990). Serum neopterin and interleukin-6 levels in chronic fatigue syndrome. *Journal of Infectious Diseases* 162:1412-1413.

Chao CC, Hu S, Ehrlich L, Peterson PK. (1995). Interleukin-1 and tumor necrosis factor-alpha syndergistically mediate neurotoxicity: Involvement of nitric oxide and of N-methyl-D-aspartate receptors. *Brain, Behavior and Immunity* 9:355.

Chao CC, Janoff EN, Hu S, Thomas K, Gallagher M, Tsang M, Peterson PK. (1991). Altered cytokine release in peripheral blood mononuclear cell cultures from patients with the chronic fatigue syndrome. *Cytokine* 3:292-298.

Cheney PR, Dorman SE, Bell DS. (1989). Interleukin-2 and the chronic fatigue syndrome. *Annals of Internal Medicine* 110(4):321.

Chester AC, Levine PH. (1994). Concurrent sick building syndrome and chronic fatigue syndrome. *Clinical Infectious Diseases* 18(Suppl. 1):S43-S48.

Chia JK, Chia LY. (1999). Chronic Chlamydia pneumoniae infection: A treatable cause of chronic fatigue syndrome. *Clinical Infectious Diseases* 29(2):452-453.

Chiu WT, Kao TY, Lin MT. (1995). Interleukin-1 receptor antagonist increases survival in rat heatstroke by reducing hypothalamic serotonin release. *Neurosciences Letters* 202:233.

Choppa PC, Vojdani A, Tagle C, Andrin R, Magtoto L. (1998). Multiplex PCR for the detection of *Mycoplasma fermentans, M. hominis* and *M. penetrans* in cell cultures and blood samples of patients with chronic fatigue syndrome. *Molecular and Cellular Probes* 12(5):301-308.

Ciampolillo A, Marini V, Mirakian R, Buscema M, Schulz T, Pujol-Borrel R, Bottazzo GF. (1989). Retrovirus-like sequences in Graves disease: Implications for human autoimmunity. *Lancet* 1(8647):1096-1110.

Cleare AJ, Heap E, Mahli GS, Wessely S, O'Keane V, Miell J. (1999). Low-dose hydrocortisone in chronic fatigue syndrome: Focus on the hypothalamic-pituitary-adrenal axis. *Functional Neurology* 14(1):3-11.

Cleare AJ, Sookdeo SS, Jones J, O'Keane V, Miell JP. (2000). Integrity of the growth hormone/insulin-like growth factor system is maintained in patients with chronic fatigue syndrome. *Journal of Clinical Endocrinology and Metabolism* 85(4):1433-1439.

Cohen N, Stempel C, Colombe B. (1990). Soluble interleukin-2 receptor: Detection and potential role in organ transplantation. *Clinical Immunology Newsletter* 10(12):175.

Cohen S, Tyrrell DA, Smith AP. (1991). Psychological stress and susceptibility to the common cold. *New England Journal of Medicine* 325(9):606-612.

Conti F, Magrini L, Priori R, Valesini G, Bonini S. (1996). Eosinophil cationic protein serum levels and allergy in chronic fatigue syndrome. *Allergy* 51(2):124-127.

Corrigan CJ, Hamid Q, North J, Barkans J, Moqbel R, Durham S, Gemou-Engesaeth V, Kay AB. (1995). Peripheral blood CD4 but not CD8 T-lymphocytes in patients with exacerbation of asthma transcribe and translate messenger RNA encoding cytokines which prolong eosinophil survival in the context of a Th2-type pattern: Effect of glucocorticoid therapy. *American Journal of Respiratory Cellular and Molecular Biology* 12(5):567-578.

Cuende JI, Civeira P, Diez N, Prieto J. (1997). High prevalence without reactivation of herpes virus 6 in subjects with chronic fatigue syndrome. *Anales de Medicina Interna* 14(9):441-444.

Cupp MJ. (1999). Herbal remedies: Adverse effects and drug interactions. *American Family Physician* 59(5):1239-1245.

Dalakas MC, Mock V, Hawkins MJ. (1998). Fatigue: Definitions, mechanisms, and paradigms for study. *Seminars in Oncology* 25(1 Suppl. 1):48-53.

Dang H, Dauphinée MJ, Talal N, Garry RF, Seibold JR, Medsger TA Jr, Alexander S, Feghali CA. (1991). Serum antibody to retroviral gag proteins in systemic sclerosis. *Arthritis and Rheumatism* 34(10):1336-1337.

Davis JM, Weaver JA, Kohut ML, Colbert LH, Ghaffar A, Mayer EP. (1998). Immune system activation and fatigue during treadmill running: Role of interferon. *Medicine and Science in Sports and Exercise* 30(6):863-868.

Daynes RA, Araneo BA. (1989). Contrasting effects of glucocorticoids on the capacity of T cells to produce the growth factors interleukin 2 and interleukin 4. *European Journal of Immunology* 19(12):2319-2325.

Daynes RA, Araneo BA, Dowell TA, Huang K, Dudley D. (1990). Regulation of murine lymphokine production in vivo. III. The lymphoid tissue microenvironment exerts regulatory influences over T helper cell function. *Journal of Experimental Medicine* 171(4):979-996.

Daynes RA, Araneo BA, Ershler WB, Maloney C, Li GZ, Ryu SY. (1993). Altered regulation of IL-6 production with normal aging. Possible linkage to the age-associated decline in dehydroepiandrosterone and its sulfated derivative. *Journal of Immunology* 150(12):5219-5230.

Daynes RA, Araneo BA, Hennebold J, Enioutina E, Mu HH. (1995). Steroids as regulators of the mammalian immune response. *Journal of Investigative Dermatology* 105:14S-19S.

Daynes RA, Meikle AW, Araneo BA. (1991). Locally active steroid hormones may facilitate compartmentalization of immunity by regulating the types of lymphokines produced by helper T cells. *Research in Immunology* 142(1):40-45.

De Becker P, De Meirleir K, Joos E, Campine I, Van Steenberge E, Smitz J, Velkeniers B. (1999). Dehydroepiandrosterone (DHEA) response to i.v. ACTH in patients with chronic fatigue syndrome. *Hormone and Metabolism Research* 31(1):18-21.

DeFreitas E, Hilliand B, Cheney P, Bell D, Kiggundu E, Sankey D, Wroblewska Z, Palladino M, Woodward JP, Koprowski H. (1991). Retroviral sequences related to human T-lymphotropic virus type II in patients with chronic fatigue immune dysfunction syndrome. *Proceedings of the National Academy of Sciences of the United States of America* 88(7):2922-2926.

Dejana E, Brenario F, Erroi A, Bussolino F, Mussoni L, Gramse M, Pintucci G, Casali B, Dinarello CA, VanDamme J. (1987). Modulation of endothelial cell function by different molecular species of interleukin-1. *Blood* 69:635-699.

Demitrack MA. (1997). Neuroendocrine correlates of chronic fatigue syndrome: A brief review. *Journal of Psychiatric Research* 31(1):69-82.

Demitrack MA. (1998). Neuroendocrine aspects of chronic fatigue syndrome: A commentary. *American Journal of Medicine* 105(3A):11S-14S.

Demitrack MA, Crofford LJ. (1998). Evidence for and pathophysiologic implications of hypothalamic-pituitary-adrenal axis dysregulation in fibromyalgia and chronic fatigue syndrome. *Annals of the New York Academy of Sciences* 840:684-697.

De Souza EB. (1993). Corticotropin-releasing factor and interleukin-1 receptors in the brain-endocrine-immune axis: Role in stress response and infection. *Annals of the New York Academy of Sciences* 697:9-27.

Diamantis I. (1996). A case from practice (343). Chronic fatigue syndrome following Lyme borreliosis. *Schweizerische Rundschau für Medizin Praxis* 85(9):287-288.

Dinan TG, Majeed T, Lavelle E, Scott LV, Berti C, Behan P. (1997). Blunted serotonin-mediated activation of the hypothalamic-pituitary-adrenal axis in chronic fatigue syndrome. *Psychoneuroendocrinology* 22(4):261-267.

Dinarello CA. (1991). Interleukin-1 and interleukin-1 antagonism. *Blood* 77(8):1627-1652.

Dinarello C. (1992). Interleukin-1 and tumor necrosis factor: Effector cytokines in autoimmune diseases. *Seminars in Immunology* 4(3):133-145.

Drancourt M, Levy MG. (1990). Rickettsial Infection. *8th Congress of the American Rickettsial Society.*

Dreisbach AW, Hendrickson T, Beezhold D, Riesenberg LA, Sklar AH. (1998). Elevated levels of tumor necrosis factor alpha in postdialysis fatigue. *International Journal of Artificial Organs* 21(2):83-86.

DuBois RE. (1986). Gamma globulin therapy for chronic mononucleosis syndrome. *AIDS Research and Human Retroviruses* 2(1):S191-S195.

Elenkov IJ, Wilder RL, Chrousos GP, Vizi ES. (2000). The sympathetic nerve—An integrative interface between two supersystems: The brain and the immune system. *Pharmacological Reviews* 52(4):595-638.

Ellenbogen C. (1997). Lyme disease. Shift the paradigm. *Archives of Family Medicine* 6(2):191-195.

Emery P, Gentry KC, Mackay IR, Muirden KD, Rowley M. (1987). Deficiency of the suppressor inducer subset of T lymphocytes in rheumatoid arthritis. *Arthritis and Rheumatism* 30: 849-856.

Evengard B, Briese T, Lindh G, Lee S, Lipkin WI. (1999). Absence of evidence of Borna disease virus infection in Swedish patients with chronic fatigue syndrome. *Journal of Neurovirology* 5(5):495-499.

Fiore G, Giacovazzo F, Giacovazzo M. (1997). Three cases of dermatomyositis erroneously diagnosed as "chronic fatigue syndrome." *European Reviews of Medical and Pharmacological Sciences* 1(6):193-195.

Fischer A, Konig W. (1991). Influence of cytokines and cellular interactions on the glucocorticoid-induced Ig (E, G, A, M) synthesis of peripheral blood mononuclear cells. *Immunology* 74(2):228-233.

Fletcher MA, Azen S, Adesberg B, Gjerset G, Hassett J, Kaplan J, Niland JC, Odom-Maryon T, Parker JW, Stites DP, et al. (1989). Immunophenotyping in a multicenter study: The transfusion safety experience. *Clinical Immunology and Immunopathology* 52:38-47.

Fletcher M, Goldstein AL. (1987). Recent advances in the understanding of the biochemistry and clinical pharmacology of interelukin-2. *Lymphokine Research* 1:45-57.

Fletcher MA, Maher K, Patarca-Montero R, Klimas N. (2000). Comparative analysis of lymphocytes in lymph nodes and peripheral blood of patients with chronic fatigue syndrome. *Journal of Chronic Fatigue Syndrome* 7(3):65-75.

Fohlman J, Friman G, Tuvemo T. (1997). Enterovirus infections in new disguise. *Lakartidningen* 94(28-29):2555-2560.

Foley FW, Traugott U, LaRocca NG, Smith CR, Perlman KR, Caruso LS, Scheinberg LC. (1992). A prospective study of depression and immune dysregulation in multiple sclerosis. *Archives of Neurology* 49(3):238-244.

Franco E, Kawa-Ha K, Doi S, Yumura K, Murata M, Ishihara S, Tawa A, Yabuuchi H. (1987). Remarkable depression of CD4+2H4+ T cells in severe chronic active Epstein-Barr virus infection. *Scandinavian Journal of Immunology* 26:769-773.

Friedman TC, Adesanya A, Poland RE. (1999). Low-dose hydrocortisone for chronic fatigue syndrome. *Journal of the American Medical Association* 281(20):1888-1889.

Fuchs D, Baier-Bitterlich G, Wachter H. (1995). Nitric oxide and AIDS dementia. *New England Journal of Medicine* 333(8):521-522.

Fuchs D, Moller AA, Reibnegger G, Stockle E, Werner ER, Wachter H. (1990). Decreased serum tryptophan in patients with HIV-1 infection correlates with increased serum neopterin and with neurologic/psychiatric symptoms. *Journal of the Acquired Immune Deficiency Syndrome* 3(9):873-876.

Fuchs D, Muur C, Reibnegger G, Weiss G, Werner ER, Werner-Felmayer G, Wachter H. (1994). Nitric oxide synthase and antimicrobial armature of human macrophages. *Journal of Infectious Diseases* 169:224.

Fukuda K, Straus SE, Hickie I, Sharpe MC, Dobbins JG, Komaroff A. (1994). International CFS Study Group. The Chronic Fatigue Syndrome: A comprehensive approach to its definition and study. *Annals of Internal Medicine* 121:953-959.

Galbraith DN, Nairn C, Clements GB. (1997). Evidence for enteroviral persistence in humans. *Journal of General Virology* 78(Pt. 2):307-312.

Gama Sosa MA, De Gasperi R, Patarca R, Fletcher MA, Kolodny EH. (1997). Antisulfatide IgG antibodies recognize HIV proteins. *Journal of Acquired Immune Deficiency Syndromes and Human Retrovirology* 15:83-90.

Garg M, Bondade S. (1993). Reversal of age-associated decline in immune response to Pnu-immune vaccine by supplementation with the steroid hormone dehydroepiandrosterone. *Infection and Immunity* 61(5):2238-2241.

Garry RF, Fermin CD, Hart DJ, Alexander SS, Donehower LA, Luo-Zhang H. (1990). Detection of a human intracisternal A-type retroviral particle antigenically related to HIV. *Science* 250(4894):1127-1129.

Gaudino EA, Coyle PK, Krupp LB. (1997). Post-Lyme syndrome and chronic fatigue syndrome. Neuropsychiatric similarities and differences. *Archives of Neurology* 54(11):1372-1376.

Glaser R, Kiecolt-Glaser JK. (1998). Stress-associated immune modulation: Relevance to viral infections and chronic fatigue syndrome. *American Journal of Medicine* 105(3A):35S-42S.

Glaser R, Lafuse WP, Bonneau RH, Atkinson C, Kiecolt-Glaser JK. (1993). Stress-associated modulation of proto-oncogene expression in human peripheral blood leukocytes. *Behavioral Neurosciences* 107(3):525-529.

Glaser R, Rabin B, Chesney M, Cohen S, Natelson B. (1999). Stress-associated immune modulation: Implications for infectious diseases? *Journal of the American Medical Association* 281(24):2268-2270.

Gold D, Bowden R, Sixbey J, Riggs R, Katon WJ, Ashley R, Obrigewitch RM, Corey L. (1990). Chronic fatigue: A prospective clinical and virologic study. *Journal of the American Medical Association* 264(1):48-53.

Goldie AS, Fearon KCH, Ross JA, Barclay R, Jackson RE, Grant IS, Ramsay G, Blyth AS, Howie JC. The Sepsis Intervention Group. (1995). Natural cytokine antagonists and endogenous antiendotoxin core antibodies in sepsis syndrome. *Journal of the American Medical Association* 274:172-177.

Goujon E, Parnet P, Cremona S, Dantzer R. (1995). Endogenous glucocorticoids down regulate central effects of interleukin-1 beta on body temperature and behaviour in mice. *Brain Research* 702:173.

Goujon E, Parnet P, Laye S, Combe C, Kelley KW, Dantzer R. (1995). Stress downregulates lipopolysaccharide-induced expression of proinflammatory cytokines in the spleen, pituitary, and brain of mice. *Brain, Behavior and Immunity* 9:292.

Griffin DE. (1991). Immunologic abnormalities accompanying acute and chronic viral infections. *Review of Infectious Diseases* 13(1):S129-S133.

Griffin WST, Stanley LC, Ling C, White L, MacLeod V, Perrot LJ, White CL, Araoz C. (1989). Brain interleukin 1 and S-100 immunoreactivity are elevated in Down's syndrome and Alzheimer's disease. *Proceedings of the National Academy of Sciences of the United States of America* 86:7611-7615.

Guida L, O'Hehir RE, Hawrylowicz CM. (1994). Synergy between dexamethasone and interleukin-5 for the induction of major histocompatibility complex class II expression by human peripheral blood eosinophils. *Blood* 84(8):2733-2740.

Gulick T, Chung MK, Pieper SJ, Lange LG, Schreiner GF. (1989). Interleukin-1 and tumor necrosis factor inhibit cardiac myocyte beta-adrenergic responsiveness. *Proceedings of the National Academy of Sciences of the United States of America* 8(17):6753-6757.

Gunn W, Komaroff A, Levine S, Connell D. (1997). Multilab retrovirus test results for CFS patients from 3 different geographical areas. *Mortality and Morbidity Weekly Report* 1 ff.

Gupta S, Aggarwal S, See D, Starr A. (1997). Cytokine production by adherent and non-adherent mononuclear cells in chronic fatigue syndrome. *Journal of Psychiatric Research* 31(1):149-156.

Gupta S, Aggarwal S, Starr A. (1999). Increased production of interleukin-6 by adherent and non-adherent mononuclear cells during "natural fatigue" but not following "experimental fatigue" in patients with chronic fatigue syndrome. *International Journal of Molecular Medicine* 3(2):209-213.

Gupta S, Vayuvegula B. (1991). A comprehensive immunological analysis in chronic fatigue syndrome. *Scandinavian Journal of Immunology* 33(3):319-327.

Hamblin TJ, Hussain J, Akbar AN, Tang YC, Smith JL, Jones DB. (1983). Immunological reason for chronic ill health after infectious mononucleosis. *British Medical Journal* 287:85-88.

Hassan IS, Bannister BA, Akbar A, Weir W, Bofill M. (1998). A study of the immunology of the chronic fatigue syndrome: Correlation of immunologic markers to health dysfunction. *Clinical Immunology and Immunopathology* 87(1):60-67.

Hayes R, Chalmers SA, Nikolic-Paterson DJ, Atkins RC, Hedger MP. (1996). Secretion of bioactive interleukin 1 by rat testicular macrophages in vitro. *Journal of Andrology* 17:41.

Hebert TB, Cohen S. (1993). Depression and immunity: A meta-analytic review. *Psychology Bulletin* 113:472-486.

Heim C, Ehlert U, Hellhammer DH. (2000). The potential role of hypocortisolism in the pathophysiology of stress-related bodily disorders. *Psychoneuroendocrinology* 25(1):1-35.

Helder L, Wagner S, Keller R, Klimas N, Antoni M. (1998). Markers of immune activation are associated with psychological distress in patients with CFS. Abstract, IV AACFS meeting, Cambridge, MA.

Hellinger WC, Smith TF, Van Scoy RE, Spidzor PG, Forgacs P, Edson RS. (1988). Chronic fatigue syndrome and diagnostic utility of antibody to Epstein-Barr virus early antigen. *Journal of the American Medical Association* 260:971-973.

Hennessy T. (1994). Nightingale's birthday: A comprehensive approach. *Annales Internationales de Medécine* 121:953-959.

Herberman RB. (1991). Sources of confounding in immunologic data. *Review of Infectious Diseases* 13(1):S84-S86.

Hernandez-Pando R, Rook GA. (1994). The role of TNF-alpha in T-cell mediated inflammation depends on the Th1/Th2 cytokine balance. *Immunology* 82(4):591-595.

Heyes MP, Saito K, Milstein S, Schiff SJ. (1995). Quinolinic acid in tumors, hemorrhage and bacterial infections of the central nervous system in children. *Journal of Neurological Sciences* 133(1-2):112-118.

Hilgers A, Frank J. (1996). Chronic fatigue syndrome: Evaluation of a 30-criteria-score and correlation with immune activation. *Journal of Chronic Fatigue Syndrome* 2(4):35-47.

Hill WM. (1996). Are echoviruses still orphan? *British Journal of Biomedical Sciences* 53(3):221-226.

Holden RJ, Mooney PA. (1995). Interleukin-1 beta: A common cause of Alzheimer's disease and diabetes mellitus. *Medical Hypotheses* 45:559.

Holmes GP, Kaplan JE, Gantz NM, Komaroff AL, Schonberger LB, Straus SE, Jones JF, Dubois RE, Cunningham-Rundles C, Pahwa S, et al. (1988). Chronic fatigue syndrome: A working case definition. *Annals of Internal Medicine* 108(3):387-389.

Holmes MJ, Diack DS, Easingwood A, Cross JP, Carlisle B. (1997). Electron microscope immunocytological profiles in chronic fatigue syndrome. *Journal of Psychiatric Research* 31(1):115-122.

Holsboer F, Von Bardeleben U, Gerken A, Stalla GK, Muller OA. (1984). Blunted corticotropin and normal cortisol response to human corticotropin-releasing factor in depression. *New England Journal of Medicine* 311(17):1127-1135.

Ho-Yen DO, Carrington D, Armstrong AA. (1988). Myalgic encephalomyelitis and alpha-interferon. *Lancet* 1:125.

Hudson M, Cleare AJ. (1999). The 1 microg short synacthen test in chronic fatigue syndrome. *Clinical Endocrinology* 51(5):625-630.

Hughes TK, Fulep E, Juelich T, Smith EM, Stanton GJ. (1995). Modulation of immune responses by anabolic androgenic steroids. *International Journal of Immunopharmacology* 17:857.

Huyser BA, Parker JC, Thoreson R, Smarr KL, Johnson JC, Hoffman R. (1998). Predictors of subjective fatigue among individuals with rheumatoid arthritis. *Arthritis and Rheumatism* 41(12):2230-2237.

Irwin M. (1993). Stress-induced immune suppression. Role of the autonomic nervous system. *Annals of the New York Academy of Sciences* 697:203-218.

Irwin M, Caldwell C, Smith TL, Brown S, Schuckit MA, Gillin C. (1990). Major depressive disorder, alcoholism, and reduced natural killer cell cytotoxicity. *Archives of General Psychiatry* 47:713-719.

Irwin M, Patterson T, Smith TL, Caldwell C, Brown SA, Gillin JC, Grant I. (1990). Reduction of immune function in life stress and depression. *Biological Psychiatry* 27:222-230.

Itoh Y, Hamada H, Imai T, Saki T, Igarashi T, Yuge K, Fukunaga Y, Yamamoto M. (1997). Antinuclear antibodies in children with chronic nonspecific complaints. *Autoimmunity* 25(4):243-250.

Iwagaki H, Hizuta A, Tanaka N, Orita K. (1995). Decreased serum tryptophan in patients with cancer cachexia correlates with increased serum neopterin. *Immunological Investigations* 24(3):467-478.

Jackson RA, Haynes BF, Burch WM, Shimizu K, Bowring MA, Eisenbarth GS. (1984). Ia+ T cells in new onset Grave's disease. *Journal of Clinical Endocrinology and Metabolism* 59:187-190.

Jacobson SK, Daly JS, Thorne GM, McIntosh K. (1997). Chronic parvovirus B19 infection resulting in chronic fatigue syndrome: Case history and review. *Clinical Infectious Diseases* 24(6):1048-1051.

Jadin CL. (1998). The Rickettsial approach of CFS. *The Clinical and Scientific Basis of CFS*. TK Roberts (Ed.) University of Newcastle, Australia, pp. 200-213.

Jadin CL. (1999). The Rickettsial approach of CFS. *CFS Manly Conference,* Australia, February.

Jadin CL. (2000). Common clinical and biological windows on CFS and Rickettsial diseases. *Journal of Chronic Fatigue Syndrome* 6(3/4):133-145.

Jadin JB. (1953). Origine des maladies Rickettsiennes. *Annales de la Societé Belge de Medécine Tropicale* 3:1 ff.

Jadin JG. (1962). Au sujet des maladies Rickettsiennes. *Annales de la Societé Belge de Medécine Tropicale* 3:321.

Jeffcoate WJ. (1999). Chronic fatigue syndrome and functional hyproadrenia-fighting vainly the old ennui. *Lancet* 353(9151):424-425.

Jones DB, Armstrong NW. (1995). Coxsackievirus and diabetes revisited. *Nature Medicine* 1:284.

Jones J. (1991). Serologic and immunologic responses in chronic fatigue syndrome with emphasis on the Epstein-Barr virus. *Reviews of Infectious Diseases* 13(1):S26-S31.

Jones JF, Ray CG, Minnich LL, Hick MJ, Kibler R, Lucus DO. (1985). Evidence for active Epstein-Barr virus infection in patients with persistent unexplained illnesses; elevated anti-early antigen antibodies. *Annals of Internal Medicine* 102:1-7.

Jones JF, Straus SE. (1987). Chronic Epstein-Barr virus infection. *Annual Reviews of Medicine* 38:195-209.

Jones SD, Koh WH, Steiner A, Garrett SL, Calin A. (1996). Fatigue in ankylosing spondylitis: Its prevalence and relationship to disease activity, sleep, and other factors. *Journal of Rheumatology* 23(3):487-490.

Jones TH, Wadler S, Hupart KH. (1998). Endocrine-mediated mechanisms of fatigue during treatment with interferon-alpha. *Seminars in Oncology* 25(1 Suppl. 1):54-63.

Kaslow JE, Rucker L, Onishi R. (1989). Liver extract-folic acid-cyanocobalamin vs. placebo for chronic fatigue syndrome. *Archives of Internal Medicine* 149:2501-2503.

Kavelaars A, Kuis W, Knook L, Sinnema G, Heijnen CJ. (2000). Disturbed neuroendocrine-immune interactions in chronic fatigue syndrome. *Journal of Clinical Endocrinology and Metabolism* 85(2):692-696.

Keller RH, Lane JL, Klimas N, Reiter WM, Fletcher MA, van Riel F, Morgan R. (1994). Association between HLA class II antigens and the chronic fatigue immune dysfunction syndrome. *Clinical Infectious Diseases* 18(Suppl. 1):S154-S156.

Kelly-Williams S, Zmijewski M, Tomaszewski E. (1989). Lymphocyte subpopulations in 'normal' lymph nodes harvested from cadavers. *Laboratory Medicine* 20:487-490.

Kibler R, Lucas DO, Hicks M, Poulos BT. Jones JF. (1985). Immune function in chronic active Epstein-Barr virus infection. *Journal of Clinical Immunology* 5:46-54.

Kitani T, Kuratsune H, Fuke I, Nakamura Y, Nakaya T, Asahi S, Tobiume M, Yamaguti M, Machii T, Inagi R, Yamanishi K, Ikuta K. (1996). Possible correlation between Borna disease virus infection and Japanese patients with chronic fatigue syndrome. *Microbiology and Immunology* 40(6):459-462.

Klimas NG. (1992). Clinical impact of adoptive therapy with purified CD8 cells in HIV infection. *Seminars in Hematology* 29:40-43.

Klimas NG, Fletcher MA. (1995). Chronic fatigue syndrome. *Current Opinion in Infectious Diseases* 8:145-148.

Klimas NG, Fletcher MA. (1999). Alteration of type 1/type 2 cytokine pattern following adoptive immunotherapy of patients with chronic fatigue syndrome (CFS) using autologous ex vivo expanded lymph node cells. Abstract, II International Conf. CFS, Brussels.

Klimas NG, Fletcher MA, Walling J, Garcia-Morales R, Patarca R, Moody D, Okarma T. (1993). Ex vivo CD8 lymphocyte activation, expansion and reinfusion into donors with rIL-2—a phase I study. In *Septieme Colloque des Cent Gardes: Retroviruses of Human AIDS and Related Animal Disease,* M. Girard and L. Valette (Eds.), pp. 285-290, Paris, France.

Klimas NG, Morgan R, Salvato F, van Riel F, Millon C, Fletcher MA. (1992). Chronic fatigue syndrome and psychoneuroimmunology. In *Stress and Disease Progression: Perspectives in Behavioral Medicine,* N Schneiderman, P McCabe, A Baum (Eds.). Lawrence Erlbaum, Assoc., Hillsdale, NJ, pp. 121-137.

Klimas NG, Patarca-Montero R, Maher K, Smith M, Bathe O, Fletcher MA. (2000). Clinical and immunologic effects of autologous lymph node cell transplant in chronic fatigue syndrome. *Journal of Chronic Fatigue Syndrome* 8(1):39-55.

Klimas NG, Patarca R, Maher K, Smith M, Jin X-Q, Huang H-S, Walling J, Gamber C, Fletcher MA. (1994). Immunomodulation with autologous, ex vivo manipulated cytotoxic T lymphocytes in HIV-1 disease. *Clinical Immunology Newsletter* 14:101-105.

Klimas NG, Patarca R, Perez G, Garcia-Morales R, Schultz D, Schabel J, Fletcher MA. (1992). Distinctive immune abnormalities in a patient with procainamide-induced lupus and serositis. *American Journal of Medical Sciences* 303(2):1-6.

Klimas NG, Patarca R, Walling J, Garcia R, Mayer V, Albarracin C, Moody D, Okarma T, Fletcher MA. (1994). Changes in the clinical and immunological stati of AIDS patients upon adoptive therapy with activated autologous CD8+ T cells and interleukin-2 infusion. *Journal of Acquired Immune Deficiency Syndromes* 8:1073-1081.

Klimas N, Salvato F, Morgan R, Fletcher MA. (1990). Immunologic abnormalities in chronic fatigue syndrome. *Journal of Clinical Microbiology* 28(6):1403-1410.

Knop J, Stremer R, Nauman C, deMaeyer E, Macher M. (1982). Interferon inhibits the suppressor T cell response of delayed hypersensitivity. *Nature* 296:757-759.

Koide J. (1985). Functional property of Ia-positive T cells in peripheral blood from patients with systemic lupus erythematosus. *Scandinavian Journal of Immunology* 22:577-584.

Kokia E, Ben-Shlomo I, Adashi EY. (1995). The ovarian action of interleukin-1 is receptor mediated: Reversal by a naturally occurring interleukin-1 receptor antagonist. *Fertility and Sterility* 63:176.

Komaroff AL, Geiger AM, Wormsley S. (1988). IgG subclass deficiencies in chronic fatigue syndrome. *Lancet* 1:1288-1289.

Konstantinov K, von Mikecz A, Buchwald D, Jones J, Gerace L, Tan EM. (1996). Autoantibodies to nuclear antigens in chronic fatigue syndrome. *Journal of Clinical Investigation* 98(8):1888-1896.

Korszun A., Papadopoulos E, Demitrack M, Engleberg C, Crofford L. (1998). The relationship between temporomandibular disorders and stress-associated syndromes. *Oral Surgery, Oral Medicine, Oral Pathology, Oral Radiology, and Endodontics* 86(4):416-420.

Kriegler M, Perez C, DeFay K, Albert I, Lu SD. (1988). A novel form of TNF-cachectin in a cell surface cytotoxic transmembrane protein: Ramifications for the complex physiology of TNF. *Cell* 53:45-53.

Kubera M, Symbirtsev A, Basta-Kaim A, Borycz J, Roman A, Papp M, Claesson M. (1996). Effect of chronic treatment with imipramine on interleukin 1 and interleukin 2 production by splenocytes obtained from rats subjected to a chronic mild stress model of depression. *Polish Journal of Pharmacology* 48:503.

Kuehn R, Rajewsky K, Mueller W. (1991). Generation and analysis of interleukin-4 deficient mice. *Science* 254:713-716.

Lagaye S, Vexiau P, Morozov V, Guenebaut-Claudet V, Tobaly-Tapiero J, Canivet M, Cathelineau G, Peries J, Emanoil-Ravier R. (1992). Human spumaretrovirus-related sequences in the DNA of leukocytes from patients with Graves disease. *Proceedings of the National Academy of Sciences of the United States of America* 89(21):10070-10074.

Lahita RG. (1982). Sex hormones and immunity. In *Basic and Clinical Immunology,* Stites DP, Stobo JD, Fudenberg HH (Eds.). Los Altos, CA: Lange, pp. 293-294.

LaManca JJ, Sisto SA, Zhou XD, Ottenweller JE, Cook S, Peckerman A, Zhang Q, Denny TN, Gause WC, Natelson BH. (1999). Immunological response in chronic fatigue syndrome following a graded exercise test to exhaustion. *Journal of Clinical Immunology* 19(2):135-142.

Landay AL, Jessop C, Lennette ET, Levy JA. (1991). Chronic fatigue syndrome: Clinical condition associated with immune activation. *Lancet* 338:707-712.

Lechin F, van der Dijs B, Acosta E, Gomez F, Lechin E, Arocha L. (1983). Distal colon motility and clinical parameters in depression. *Journal of Affective Disorders* 5:19-26.

Lechin F, van der Dijs B, Amat J, Lechin M. (1989). Central neuronal pathways involved in depressive syndrome: Experimental findings. In *Neurochemistry and Clinical Disorders: Circuitry of Some Psychiatric and Psychosomatic Syndromes,* Lechin F, van der Dijs B (Eds.). Boca Raton, FL: CC Press, pp. 65-89.

Lechin F, van der Dijs B, Gomez F, Arocha L, Acosta E, Lechin E. (1983). Distal colon motility as a predictor of antidepressant response to fenfluramine, imipramine and clomipramine. *Journal of Affective Disorders* 5:27-35.

Lechin F, van der Dijs B, Jakubowicz D, Camero RE, Lechin S, Villa S, Reinfeld B, Lechin ME. (1987). Role of stress in the exacerbation of chronic illness: Effects of clonidine administration on blood pressure and plasma norepinephrine, cortisol, growth hormone and prolactin concentrations. *Psychoneuroendocrinology* 12(2):117-129.

Lechin F, van der Dijs B, Jakubowicz D, Camero RE, Villa S, Arocha L, Lechin AE. (1985). Effects of clonidine on blood pressure, noradrenaline, cortisol, growth hormone and prolactin plasma levels in low and high intestinal tone depressed patients. *Neuroendocrinology* 41(2):156-162.

Lechin F, van der Dijs B, Lechin A, Orozco B, Lechin M, Baez S, Rada I, Leon G, Acosta E. (1994). Plasma neurotransmitters and cortisol in chronic illness: Role of stress. *Journal of Medicine* 25:181-192.

Lee SC, Dickson DW, Brosnan CF. (1995). Interleukin-1, nitric oxide and reactive astrocytes. *Brain, Behavior and Immunity* 9:345.

Levine PH, Whiteside TL, Friberg D, Bryant J, Colclough G, Herberman RB. (1998). Dysfunction of natural killer activity in a family with chronic fatigue syndrome. *Clinical Immunology and Immunopathology* 88(1):96-104.

Levine S. (1999). Borna disease virus proteins in patients with CFS. *Journal of Chronic Fatigue Syndrome* 5(3/4):199-206.

Levy JA, Greenspan D, Ferro F, Lennette ET. (1990). Frequent isolation of HHV-6 from saliva and high seroprevalence of the virus in the population. *Lancet* 335:1047-1050.

Lijima H, Sun S, Cyong JC, Jyonouchi H. (1999). Juzen-taiho-to, a Japanese herbal medicine, modulates type 1 and type 2 T-cell responses in old BALB/c mice. *American Journal of Chinese Medicine* 27(2):191-203.

Lindal E, Bergmann S, Thorlacius S, Stefansson JG. (1997). Anxiety disorders: A result of long-term chronic fatigue—The psychiatric characteristics of the sufferers of Iceland disease. *Acta Neurologica Scandinavica* 96(3):158-162.

Linde A, Andersson B, Svenson SB, Ahrne H, Carlsson M, Forsberg P, Hugo H, Karstop A, Lenkei R, Lindwall A, et al. (1992). Serum levels of lymphokines and soluble cellular receptors in primary EBV infection and in patients with chronic fatigue syndrome. *Journal of Infectious Diseases* 165:994-1000.

Linde A, Hammarstrom L, Smith CIE. (1988). IgG subclass deficiency and chronic fatigue syndrome. *Lancet* 1:885-886.

Lindelman C, Mellstedt H, Biverfeld P. (1983). Blood and lymph node T-lymphocyte subsets in non-Hodgkin lymphomas. *Scandinavian Journal of Haematology* 30:68-78.

Lindh G, Samuelson A, Hedlund KO, Evengard B, Lindquist L, Ehrnst A. (1996). No findings of enteroviruses in Swedish patients with chronic fatigue syndrome. *Scandinavian Journal of Infectious Diseases* 28(3):305-307.

Lloyd A, Hanna DA, Wakefield D. (1988). Interferon and myalgic encephalomyelitis. *Lancet* 1:471.

Lloyd A, Hickie I, Hickie C, Dwyer J, Wakefield D. (1992). Cell-mediated immunity in patients with chronic fatigue syndrome, healthy controls and patients with major depression. *Clinical and Experimental Immunology* 87(1):76-79.

Lloyd A, Hickie I, Wakefield D, Boughton C, Dwyer J. (1990). A double-blind, placebo-controlled trial of intravenous immunoglobulin therapy in patients with chronic fatigue syndrome. *American Journal of Medicine* 89:561-568.

Lloyd AR, Wakefield D, Boughton CR, Dwyer JM. (1989). Immunological abnormalities in the chronic fatigue syndrome. *Medical Journal of Australia* 151:122-124.

Lusso P, Salahuddin SZ, Ablashi DV, Gallo RC, Di Marzo Veronese F, Markham PD. (1987). Diverse tropism of HBLV (human herpesvirus 6). *Lancet* 2(8561): 743.

Lutgendorf S, Antoni MH, Ironson G, Fletcher MA, Penendo F, Van Riel F, Baum A, Schneiderman N, Klimas N. (1995). Physical symptoms of chronic fatigue syndrome are exacerbated by the stress of Hurricane Andrew. *Psychosomatic Medicine* 57:310-323.

Lutgendorf S, Klimas N, Antoni M, Brickman A, Fletcher MA. (1995). Relationships of cognitive difficulties to immune measures, depression and illness burden in chronic fatigue syndrome. *Journal of Chronic Fatigue Syndrome* 1:23-41.

MacHale SM, Cavanagh JT, Bennie J, Carroll S, Goodwin GM, Lawrie SM. (1998). Diurnal variation of adrenocortical activity in chronic fatigue syndrome. *Neuropsychobiology* 38(4):213-217.

Mackay CR. (1992). Migration pathways and immunologic memory among T lymphocytes. *Seminars in Immunology* 4:51-58.

Mackay CR, Martson WL, Dudler L. (1990). Naive and memory T cells show distinct pathways of lymphocyte recirculation. *Journal of Experimental Medicine* 171:801-817.

Maes M, Vandoolaeghe E, Ranjan R, Bosmans E, Bergmans R, Desnyder R. (1995). Increased serum interleukin-1-receptor-antagonist concentrations in major depression. *Journal of Affective Disorders* 36:29.

Malkovsky M, Loveland B, North M, Asherton GL, Gao L, Ward P, Fiers W. (1987). Recombinant interleukin-2 directly augments the cytotoxicity of human monocytes. *Nature* 32(6101):262-265.

Malone JL, Simms TE, Gray GC, Wagner KF, Burge JR, Burke DS. (1990). Sources of variability in repeated T-helper lymphocyte counts from human immunodeficiency virus type 1-infected patients: Total lymphocyte count fluctuations and diurnal cycle are important. *Journal of Acquired Immune Deficiency Syndromes* 3(2):144-151.

Marcusson JA, Lindh G, Evengard B. (1999). Chronic fatigue syndrome and nickel allergy. *Contact Dermatitis* 40(5):269-272.

Marmion BP, Shannon M, Maddock I, Storm P, Penttila I. (1996). Protracted debility and fatigue after acute Q fever. *Lancet* 347(9006):977-978.

Marsh S, Kaplan M, Asano Y, Hoekzema D, Komaroff AL, Whitman JE Jr, Ablashi DV. (1996). Development and application of HHV-6 antigen capture assay for the detection of HHV-6 infections. *Journal of Virological Methods* 61(1-2): 103-112.

Martin E, Muler JV, Dionel C. (1988). Disappearance of CD4 lymphocyte circadian cycles in HIV-infected patients: Early event during asymptomatic infection. *AIDS* 2:133-134.

Martin WJ. (1996a). Genetic instability and fragmentation of a stealth viral genome. *Pathobiology* 64(1):9-17.

Martin WJ. (1996b). Severe stealth virus encephalopathy following chronic-fatigue syndrome-like illness: Clinical and histopathological features. *Pathobiology* 64 (1):1-8.

Martin WJ. (1997). Detection of RNA sequences in cultures of a stealth virus isolated from the cerebrospinal fluid of a health care worker with chronic fatigue syndrome. Case report. *Pathobiology* 65(1):57-60.

Martin WJ. (1998). Cellular sequences in stealth viruses. *Pathobiology* 66(2):53-58.

Martin WJ. (1999). Stealth adaptation of an African green monkey simian cytomegalovirus. *Experimental Molecular Pathology* 66(1):3-7.

Marwick C. (2000). International plan focuses on eradication of polio and containment of the virus. *Journal of the American Medical Association* 283(12):1553-1554.

Masuda A, Nozoe SI, Matsuyama T, Tanaka H. (1994). Psychobehavioral and immunological characteristics of adult people with chronic fatigue and patients with chronic fatigue syndrome. *Psychosomatic Medicine* 56(6):516-518.

Mauff G, Gon M. (1991). CFS in Incline Village. *Southern Association Medical Journal,* March.

Mawle AC, Nisenbaum R, Dobbins JG, Gary HE Jr, Stewart JA, Reyes M, Steele L, Schmid DS, Reeves WC. (1997). Immune responses associated with chronic fatigue syndrome: A case-control study. *Journal of Infectious Diseases* 175(1):136-141.

McAllister CG, Rapaport MH, Pickar D, Podruchny TA, Christison G, Alphs LD, Paul SM. (1989). Increased numbers of CD5+ B lymphocytes in schizophrenic patients. *Archives of General Psychiatry* 46:890-894.

McArdle A, McArdle F, Jackson MJ, Page SF, Fahal I, Edwards RH. (1996). Investigation by polymerase chain reaction of enteroviral infection in patients with chronic fatigue syndrome. *Clinical Science* 90(4):295-300.

McKenzie R, O'Fallon A, Dale J, Demitrack M, Sharma G, Deloria M, Garcia-Borreguero D, Blackwelder W, Straus SE. (1998). Low-dose hydrocortisone for treatment of chronic fatigue syndrome: A randomized controlled trial. *Journal of the American Medical Association* 280(12):1061-1066.

McRae S. (1996). Elevated serum digoxin levels in a patient taking digoxin and Siberian ginseng. *Canadian Medical Association Journal* 155(3):293-295, comment 155(9):1237.

Miller LG. (1998). Herbal medicinals: Selected clinical considerations focusing on known or potential drug-herb interactions. *Archives of Internal Medicine* 158(20):2200-2211.

Miller NA, Carmichael HA, Hall FC, Calder BD. (1991). Antibody to coxsackie B virus in diagnosing postviral fatigue syndrome. *British Medical Journal* 302:140-143.

Millon C, Salvato F, Blaney F, Morgan R, Mantero-Atienza E, Klimas NG, Fletcher MA. (1989). A psychological assessment of chronic fatigue syndrome/chronic Epstein-Barr virus patients. *Psychology and Health* 3:131-141.

Miyakoshi H, Aoki T, Mizukoshi. (1984). Acting mechanisms of Lentinan in humans. II. Enhancement of non-specific cell-mediated cytotoxicity as an interferon induced response. *International Journal of Immunopharmacology* 6:373-379.

Mizel SB. (1989). The interleukins. *FASEB Journal* 3:2379-2388.

Moldovsky H. (1989). Nonrestorative sleep and symptoms after a febrile illness in patients with fibrosis and chronic fatigue syndrome. *Journal of Rheumatology* 16(19):150-153.

Morag A, Tobi M, Ravid Z, Ravel M, Schattner A. (1982). Increased (2'-5')-oligo-a synthetase activity in patients with prolonged illness associated with serological evidence of persistent Epstein-Barr virus infection. *Lancet* 1:744.

Morales AJ, Nolan JJ, Nelson JC, Yen SS. (1994). Effects of replacement dose of dehydroepiandrosterone in men and women of advancing age. *Journal of Clinical Endocrinology and Metabolism* 78(6):1360-1367.

Morgan DA, Ruscetti FW, Gallo RC. (1976). Selective in vitro growth of T lymphocytes from normal human bone marrows. *Science* 193:1007-1008.

Morimoto C, Letvin NL, Distaso JA, Aldrich WR, Schlossman SF. (1985). The isolation and characterization of the human suppressor inducer T cell subset. *Journal of Immunology* 134(3): 1508-1512.

Morrison LJ, Behan WH, Behan PO. (1991). Changes in natural killer cell phenotype in patients with post-viral fatigue syndrome. *Clinical and Experimental Immunology* 83:441-446.

Morte S, Castilla A, Civeira M-P, Serrano M, Prieto J. (1988). Gamma-interferon and chronic fatigue syndrome. *Lancet* 2:623-624.

Morte S, Castilla A, Civeira M-P, Serrano M, Prieto J. (1989). Production of interleukin-1 by peripheral blood mononuclear cells in patients with chronic fatigue syndrome. *Journal of Infectious Diseases* 159:362.

Moss RB, Mercandetti A, Vojdani A. (1999). TNF-alpha and chronic fatigue syndrome. *Journal of Clinical Immunology* 19(5):314-316.

Mu HH, Sewell WA. (1993). Enhancement of interleukin-4 production by pertussis toxin. *Infection and Immunity* 61(7):3190-3198.

Nakaya T, Kuratsune H, Kitani T, Ikuta K. (1997). Demonstration on Borna disease virus in patients with chronic fatigue syndrome. *Nippon Rinsho—Japanese Journal of Clinical Medicine* 55(11):3064-3071.

Nakaya T, Takahashi H, Nakamura Y, Asahi S, Tobiume M, Kuratsune H, Kitani T, Yamanishi K, Ikuta K. (1996). Demonstration of Borna disease virus RNA in peripheral blood mononuclear cells derived from Japanese patients with chronic fatigue syndrome. *FEBS Letters* 378(2):145-149.

Nasralla M, Haier J, Nicolson GL. (1999). Multiple mycoplasmal infections detected in blood of patients with chronic fatigue syndrome and/or fibromyalgia syndrome. *European Journal of Clinical Microbiology and Infectious Diseases* 18(12):859-865.

Natelson BH, LaManca JJ, Denny TN, Vladutiu A, Oleske J, Hill N, Bergen MT, Korn L, Hay J. (1998). Immunologic parameters in chronic fatigue syndrome, major depression, and multiple sclerosis. *American Journal of Medicine* 105(3A):43S-49S.

Nicolson GL, Nasralla M, Franco AR, De Meierleir K, Nicolson NL, Ngwenya R, Haier J. (2000). Role of mycoplasmal infections in fatigue illnesses: Chronic fatigue and fibromyalgia syndromes, Gulf War illness, and rheumatoid arthritis. *Journal of Chronic Fatigue Syndrome* 6(3/4):23-39.

Nicolson GL, Nasralla M, Haier J. (1998). Diagnosis and treatment of mycoplasmal infections in fibromyalgia and chronic fatigue syndromes: Relationship to Gulf War illness. *Biomedical Therapy* 16:266-271.

Nilsson L, Kjellman NI, Storsaeter J, Gustafsson L, Olin P. (1996). Lack of association between pertussis vaccine and symptoms of asthma and allergy. *Journal of the American Medical Association* 275(10):760.

Nishikai M, Akiya K, Tojo T, Onoda N, Tani M, Shimizu K. (1996). "Seronegative" Sjoegren's syndrome manifested as a subset of chronic fatigue syndrome. *British Journal of Rheumatology* 35(5):471-474.

Nishikai M, Kosaka S. (1997). Incidence of antinuclear antibodies in Japanese patients with chronic fatigue syndrome. *Arthritis and Rheumatism* 40(11):2095-2097.

Nowotny N, Kolodziejek J. (2000). Human Bornaviruses and laboratory strains. *Lancet* 355(9213):1462-1463.

Odent MR, Culpin EE, Kimmel T. (1994). Pertussis vaccination and asthma: Is there a link? *Journal of the American Medical Association* 272(8):592-593.

Ogawa M, Nishiura T, Yoshimura M, Horikawa Y, Yoshida H, Okajima Y, Matsumura I, Ishikawa J, Nakao H, Tomiyama Y, Kanayama Y, Kanakura Y, Matsuzawa Y. (1998). Decreased nitric oxide-mediated natural killer cell activation in chronic fatigue syndrome. *European Journal of Clinical Investigation* 28(11):937-943.

Ojo-Amaise EA, Conley EJ, Peters JB. (1994). Decreased natural killer cell activity is associated with severity of chronic fatigue immune deficiency syndrome. *Clinical Infectious Diseases* 18:S157-S159.

Olson GB, Kanaan MN, Gersuk GM, Kelley LM, Jones JF. (1986). Correlation between allergy and persistent Epstein-Barr virus infections in chronic active Epstein-Barr virus infected patients. *Journal of Allergy and Clinical Immunology* 78(2):308-314.

Olson GB, Kanaan MN, Kelley LM, Jones JF. (1986). Specific allergen-induced Epstein-Barr nuclear antigen-positive B cells from patients with chronic active Epstein-Barr virus infections. *Journal of Allergy and Clinical Immunology* 78(2): 315-320.

Onouchi H, Muro Y, Tomita Y. (1999). Clinical features and IgG subclass distribution of anti-p80 coli antibodies. *Journal of Autoimmunity* 13(2):225-232.

Ottaviani E, Franchini A. (1995). Immune and neuroendocrine responses in molluscs: The role of cytokines. *Acta Biologica Hungarica* 46:341.

Padgett DA, Sheridan JF, Loria RM. (1995). Steroid hormone regulation of a polyclonal TH2 immune response. *Annals of the New York Academy of Sciences* 774:323-325.

Paez Pereda M, Perez Castro C, Costas M, Nahmod VE, Stalla GK, Holsboer F, Artz E. (1996). Glucocorticoids inhibit the autoregulatory induction of interleukin-1 in monocytes after endotoxin stimulation. *Neuroimmunomodulation* 3:227.

Pall ML. (2000). Elevated, sustained peroxynitrite levels as the cause of chronic fatigue syndrome. *Medical Hypotheses* 54(1):115-125.

Paris MM, Friedland IR, Ehrett S, Hickey SM, Olsen KD, Hansen E, Thonar EJ, McCracken GH Jr. (1995). Effect of interleukin-1 receptor antagonist and soluble tumor necrosis factor receptor in animal models of infection. *Journal of Infectious Diseases* 171:161.

Patarca R. (1997). Pteridines and neuroimmune function and pathology. *Journal of Chronic Fatigue Syndrome* 3(1):69-86.

Patarca R. (2000). *Concise Encyclopedia of Chronic Fatigue Syndrome.* Binghamton, NY: The Haworth Press, pp. 1 ff.

Patarca R, Fletcher MA, Klimas NG. (1992). Immunological correlates of the chronic fatigue syndrome. In *Chronic Fatigue Syndrome,* P Goodnick, NG Klimas (Eds.). Washington: American Psychiatric Press, pp. 1-21.

Patarca R, Goodkin K, Fletcher MA. (1995). Cryopreservation of peripheral blood mononuclear cells. In *Manual of Clinical Laboratory Immunology,* Rose NR, de Macario EC, Folds JD, Lane HC, Nakamura RM, (Eds.). Washington, DC: American Society of Microbiology Press, pp. 281-286.

Patarca R, Klimas NG, Garcia MN, Pons H, Fletcher MA. (1995). Dysregulated expression of soluble immune mediator receptors in a subset of patients with chronic fatigue syndrome: Categorization of patients by immune status. *Journal of Chronic Fatigue Syndrome* 1:79-94.

Patarca R, Klimas NG, Sandler D, Garcia MN, Fletcher MA. (1995). Interindividual immune status variation patterns in patients with chronic fatigue syndrome: Association with the tumor necrosis factor system and gender. *Journal of Chronic Fatigue Syndrome* 2(1):13-19.

Patarca R, Klimas NG, Walling J, Mayer V, Baum M, Yue X-S, Garcia MN, Pons H, Sandler D, Friedlander A, Page B, Lai S, Fletcher MA. (1994). CD8 T-cell immunotherapy in AIDFS: Rationale and lessons learned at the cellular and molecular biology levels. *Clinical Immunology Newsletter* 14:105-111.

Patarca R, Klimas NG, Walling J, Sandler D, Friedlander A, Jin X-Q, Garcia MN, Fletcher MA. (1995). Adoptive CD8+ T-cell immunotherapy of AIDS patients with Kaposi's sarcoma. *Critical Reviews in Oncogenesis* 6(3-6):179-234.

Patarca R, Lugtendorf S, Antoni M, Klimas NG, Fletcher MA. (1994). Dysregulated expression of tumor necrosis factor in the chronic fatigue immune dysfunction syndrome: Interrelations with cellular sources and patterns of soluble immune mediator expression. *Clinical Infectious Diseases* 18:S147-S153.

Patarca R, Sandler D, Walling J, Klimas NG, Fletcher MA. (1995). Assessment of immune mediator expression levels in biological fluids and cells: A critical appraisal. *Critical Reviews in Oncogenesis* 6(2):117-149.

Patarca-Montero R, Klimas NG, Fletcher MA. (2000). Immunotherapy of chronic fatigue syndrome: Therapeutic interventions aimed at modulating the Th1/Th2 cytokine expression balance. *Journal of Chronic Fatigue Syndrome* 8(1):3-37.

Paul WE, Ohara J. (1987). B-cell stimulatory factor-1/interleukin-4. *Annual Reviews of Immunology* 5:429-459.

Pavol MA, Meyers CA, Rexer JL, Valentine AD, Mattis PJ, Talapaz M. (1995). Pattern of neurobehavioral deficits with interferon alpha therapy for leukemia. *Neurology* 45(5):947-950.

Peakman M, Deale A, Field R, Mahalingam M, Wessely S. (1997). Clinical improvement in chronic fatigue syndrome is not associated with lymphocyte subsets of function or activation. *Clinical Immunology and Immunopathology* 82(1):83-91.

Pellegrini P, Berghella AM, Di Loreto S, Del Beato T, Di Marco F, Adorno D, Casciani CU. (1996). Cytokine contribution to the repair processes and homeostasis recovery following anoxic insult: A possible IFN-gamma-regulating role in IL-1beta neurotoxic action in physiological repair. *Neuroimmunodulation* 3:213.

Penttila IA, Harris RJ, Storm P, Haynes D, Worswick DA, Marmion BP. (1998). Cytokine dysregulation in the post-Q-fever fatigue syndrome. *Quarterly Journal of Medicine* 91(8):549-560.

Perl A, Gorevic PD, Condemi JJ, Papsidero L, Poiesz BJ, Abraham GN. (1991). Antibodies to retroviral proteins and reverse transcriptase activity in patients with essential cryoglobulinemia. *Arthritis and Rheumatism* 34(10):313-318.

Peterson PK, Shepard J, Macres M, Schenck C, Crosson J, Rechtman D, Lunie N. (1990). A controlled trial of intravenous immunoglobulin G in chronic fatigue syndrome. *American Journal of Medicine* 89(5):554-560.

Platanias LC, Vogelzang NJ. (1990). Interleukin-1: Biology, pathophysiology, and clinical prospects. *American Journal of Medicine* 89(5):621-629.

Plioplys AV. (1997). Antimuscle and anti-CNS circulating antibodies in chronic fatigue syndrome. *Neurology* 48(6):1717-1719.

Poteliakhoff A. (1998). Fatigue syndromes and the aetiology of autoimmune disease. *Journal of Chronic Fatigue Syndrome* 4(4):31-50.

Prieto J, Subira ML, Castilla A, Serrano M. (1989). Naloxone-reversible monocyte dysfunction in patients with chronic fatigue syndrome. *Scandinavian Journal of Immunology* 30(1):13-20.

Pruessner JC, Hellhammer DH, Kirschbaum C. (1999). Burnout, perceived stress, and cortisol responses to awakening. *Psychosomatic Medicine* 61(2):197-204.

Pui CH. (1989). Serum interleukin-2 receptor: Clinical and biological implications. *Leukemia* 3(5):323-327.

Rabinowe SL, Jackson RA, Dluhy RG, et al. (1984). Ia-positive T lymphocytes in recently diagnosed idiopathic Addison's disease. *American Journal of Medicine* 77:597-601.

Ramiya VK, Shang XZ, Pharis PG, Wasserfall CH, Stabler TV, Muir AB, Schatz DA, Maclaren NK. (1996). Antigen based therapies to prevent diabetes in NOD mice. *Journal of Autoimmunity* 9:349-356.

Rasmussen AK, Nielsen AH, Andersen V, Barington T, Bendtzen K, Hansen MB, Nielsen L, Pederson BK, Wiik A. (1994). Chronic fatigue syndrome—A controlled cross sectional study. *Journal of Rheumatology* 21(8):1527-1531.

Ravdin LD, Hilton E, Primeau M, Clements C, Barr WB. (1996). Memory functioning in Lyme borreliosis. *Journal of Clinical Psychiatry* 57(7):282-286.

Raven PW, Checkley SA, Taylor NF. (1995). Extra-adrenal effects of metyrapone include inhibition of the 11-oxoreductase activity of 11 beta-hydroxysteroid dehydrogenase: A model for 11-HSD I deficiency. *Clinical Endocrinology* 43(5):637-644.

Raven PW, O'Dwyer AM, Taylor NF, Checkley SA. (1996). The relationship between the effects of metyrapone treatment on depressed mood and urinary steroid profiles. *Psychoneuroendocrinology* 21(3):277-286.

Raziuddin S, Elawad ME. (1990). Immunoregulatory CD4+CD45R+ suppressor/inducer T lymphocyte subsets and impaired cell-mediated immunity in patients with Down's syndrome. *Clinical and Experimental Immunology* 79:67-71.

Read R, Spickett G, Harvey J, Edwards AJ, Larson HE. (1988). IgG1 subclass deficiency in patients with chronic fatigue syndrome. *Lancet* 1(8579):241-242.

Regland B, Zachrisson O, Stejskal V, Gottfries CG. (2000). Nickel allergy is found in a majority of women with chronic fatigue syndrome and muscle pain—And may be triggered by cigarette smoke and dietary nickel intake. *Journal of Chronic Fatigue Syndrome* 8(1):57-65.

Reinherz EL, Schlossman SF. (1981). The characterization and function of human immunoregulatory T lymphocyte subsets. *Immunology Today* 2:6975-6979.

Rettori V, Gimeno MF, Karara A, Gonzalez MC, McCann SM. (1991). Interleukin 1a inhibits prostaglandin E_2 release to suppress pulsatile release of luteinizing hormone but not follicle-stimulating hormone. *Proceedings of the National Academy of Sciences of the United States of America* 88:2763-2767.

Riemsma RP, Rasker JJ, Taal E, Griep EN, Wouters JM, Wiegman O. (1998). Fatigue in rheumatoid arthritis: The role of self-efficacy and problematic social support. *British Journal of Rheumatology* 37(10):1042-1046.

Roberts TK, McGregor NR, Dunstan RH, Donohoe M, Murdoch RN, Hope D, Zhang S, Butt HL, Watkins JA, Taylor WG. (1998). Immunological and haematological parameters in patients with chronic fatigue syndrome. *Journal of Chronic Fatigue Syndrome* 4(4):51-66.

Romain P, Schlossman S. (1984). Human T lymphocyte subsets: Functional heterogeneity and surface recognition structures. *Journal of Clinical Investigation* 74:1559-1565.

Rook GA, Hernandez-Pando R. (1996). The pathogenesis of tuberculosis. *Annual Reviews of Microbiology* 50:259-284.

Rook GA, Stanford JL. (1996). The Koch phenomenon and the immunopathology of tuberculosis. *Current Topics in Microbiology and Immunology* 215:239-262.

Rook GA, Zumla A. (1997). Gulf War syndrome: Is it due to a systemic shift in cytokine balance towards a Th2 profile? *Lancet* 349(9068):1831-1833.

Roubalova K, Roubal J, Skopovy P, Fucikova T, Domorazkova E, Vonka V. (1988). Antibody response to Epstein-Barr virus antigens in patients with chronic viral infection. *Journal of Medical Virology* 25(1):115-122.

Rowe KS. (1997). Double-blind randomized controlled trial to assess the efficacy of intravenous gammaglobulin for the management of chronic fatigue syndrome in adolescents. *Journal of Psychiatric Research* 31(1):133-147.

Rupprecht R, Hauser CA, Trapp TA, Holsboer F. (1996). Neurosteroids: Molecular mechanisms of action and psychopharmacological significance. *Journal of Steroid Biochemistry and Molecular Biology* 56(1-6):163-168.

Saito K. (1995). Biochemical studies on AIDS dementia complex—possible contribution of quinolinic acid during brain damage. *Rinsho Byori-Japanese Journal of Clinical Pathology* 43(9):891-901.

Salit IE. (1985). Sporadic postinfectious neuromyasthenia. *Canadian Medical Association Journal* 133:659-663.

Salvatore M, Morozunov M, Schnemake M, Lipkin WI and the Bornavirus study group. (1998). Borna disease virus in brains of North American and European people with schizophrenia and bipolar disorders. *Lancet* 349:1813-1814.

Sandman CA, Barron JL, Nackoul KA, Fidler PL, Goldstein J. (1992). Is there a chronic fatigue syndrome (CFS) dementia? In *The Clinical and Scientific Basis of Myalgic Encephalomyelitis/Chronic Fatigue Syndrome*, Hyde B, Levine P, Goldstein J (Eds.). Nightingale Research Foundation. Ottawa, Canada: pp. 467-479.

Sapolsky R, Rivier C, Yamamoto G, Plotsky P, Vale W. (1987). Interleukin-1 stimulates the secretion of hypothalamic corticotropin-releasing factor. *Science* 238(4826):522-524.

Sato K, Miyasaka N, Yamaoka K, Okuda M, Yata J, Nishioka K. (1987). Quantitative defect of CD4+2H4+ cells in systemic lupus erythematosus and Sjogren's syndrome. *Arthritis and Rheumatism* 30(12):1407-1411.

Sauder C, Muller A, Cubitt B, Mayer J, Steimetz J, Trabert W, Ziegler B, Wanke K, Mueller-Lantzsch N, de la Torre JC, Grasser FA. (1996). Detection of Borna disease virus (BDV) antibodies and BDV RNA psychiatric patients: Evidence of high sequence conservation of human blood-derived RNA. *Journal of Virology* 70(1):7713-7724.

Schleifer SJ, Keller SE, Bond RN, Cohen J, Stein M. (1989). Major depressive disorder: Role of age, sex, severity and hospitalization. *Archives of General Psychiatry* 46:81-87.

Schmaling KB, Jones JF. (1996). MMPI profiles of patients with chronic fatigue syndrome. *Journal of Psychosomatic Research* 40(1):67-74.

Schulte PA. (1991). Validation of biologic markers for use in research on chronic fatigue syndrome. *Review of Infectious Disease* 13:S87-S89.

Schutzer SE, Natelson BH. (1999). Absence of Borrelia burgdorferi-specific immune complexes in chronic fatigue syndrome. *Neurology* 53(6):1340-1341.

Scott LV, Burnett F, Medbak S, Dinan TG. (1998). Naloxone-mediated activation of the hypothalamic-pituitary-adrenal axis in chronic fatigue syndrome. *Psychological Medicine* 28(2):285-293.

Scott LV, Dinan TG. (1998). Urinary cortisol excretion in chronic fatigue syndrome, major depression and in health volunteers. *Journal of Affective Disorders* 47(1-3):49-54.

Scott LV, Dinan TG. (1999). The neuroendocrinology of chronic fatigue syndrome: Focus on the hypothalamic-pituitary-adrenal axis. *Functional Neurology* 14(1):3-11.

Scott LV, Medbak S, Dinan TG. (1998a). Blunted adrenocorticotropin and cortisol responses to corticotropin-releasing hormone stimulation in chronic fatigue syndrome. *Acta Psychiatrica Scandinavica* 97(6):450-457.

Scott LV, Medbak S, Dinan TG. (1998b). The low dose ACTH test in chronic fatigue syndrome and in health. *Clinical Endocrinology* 48(6):733-737.

Scott LV, Medbak S, Dinan TG. (1999). Desmopressin augments pituitary-adrenal responsivity to corticotropin-releasing hormone in subjects with chronic fatigue syndrome and in healthy volunteers. *Biological Psychiatry* 45(11):1447-1454.

Scott LV, Salahuddin F, Cooney J, Svec F, Dinan TG. (1999). Differences in adrenal steroid profile in chronic fatigue syndrome, in depression and in health. *Journal of Affective Disorders* 54(1-2):129-137.

Scott LV, The J, Reznek R, Martin A, Sohaib A, Dinan TG. (1999). Small adrenal glands in chronic fatigue syndrome: A preliminary computer tomography study. *Psychoneuroendocrinology* 24(7):759-768.

See DM, Broumand N, Sahl L, Tilles TG. (1997). In vitro effects of echinacea and ginseng on natural killer and antibody-dependent cell cytotoxicity in healthy subjects and chronic fatigue syndrome or acquired immunodeficiency syndrome patients. *Immunopharmacology* 35(3):229-235.

See DM, Cimoch P, Chou S, Chang J, Tilles J. (1998). The in vitro immunodulatory effects of glyconutrients on peripheral blood mononuclear cells of patients with chronic fatigue syndrome. *Integrative Physiological and Behavioral Science* 33(3):280-287.

See DM, Tilles JG. (1996). Alpha-interferon treatment of patients with chronic fatigue syndrome. *Immunological Investigations* 25(1-2):153-164.

Sellami S, de Beaurepaire R. (1995). Hypothalamic and thalamic sites of action of interleukin-1 beta on food intake, body temperature and pain sensitivity in the rat. *Brain Research* 694:769.

Shaheen SO, Aaby P, Hall AJ, Barker DJ, Heyes CB, Shiell AW, Goudiaby A. (1996). Measles and atopy in Guinea-Bissau. *Lancet* 347:1792-1796.

Shanks N, Francis D, Zaleman S, Meaney MJ, Anisman H. (1994). Alterations in central cathecolamines associated with immune responses in adult and aged mice. *Brain Research* 666(1):77-87.

Sharpe M, Clements A, Hawton K, Young AH, Sargent P, Cowen PJ. (1996). Increased prolactin response to buspirone in chronic fatigue syndrome. *Journal of Affective Disorders* 41(1):71-76.

Sharpe M, Hawton K, Clements A, Cowen PJ. (1997). Increased brain serotonin function in men with chronic fatigue syndrome. *British Medical Journal* 315(7101):164-165.

Shaskan EG, Brew BJ, Rosenblum M, Thompson RM, Price RW. (1992). Increased neopterin levels in brains of patients with human immunodeficiency virus type 1 infection. *Journal of Neurochemistry* 59(4):1541-1546.

Sheng WS, Hu S, Lamkin A, Peterson PK, Chao CC. (1996). Susceptibility to immunologically mediated fatigue in C57BL/6 versus BALB/c mice. *Clinical Immunology and Immunopathology* 81(2):161-167.

Shoham S, Davenne D, Cady AB, Dinarello CA, Krueger JM. (1987). Recombinant tumor necrosis factor and interleukin 1 enhance slow-wave sleep. *American Journal of Physiology* 253:R142-R149.

Silvestris F, Williams RC, Dammacco F. (1995). Autoreactivity in HIV-1 infection: The role of molecular mimicry. *Clinical Immunology and Immunopathology* 75:197-205.

Skaper SD, Facci L, Leon A. (1995). Inflammatory mediator stimulation of astrocytes and meningeal fibroblasts induces neuronal degeneration via the nitridergic pathway. *Journal of Neurochemistry* 64:266.

Smit JA, Stark JH, Myburgh JA. (1996). Induction of primate TH2 lymphokines to suppress TH1 cells. *Transplantation Proceedings* 28(2):665-666.

Sobel RA, Hafler DA, Castro EE, et al. (1988). The 2H4 (CD45R) antigen is selectively decreased in multiple sclerosis lesions. *Journal of Immunology* 140:2210-2214.

Song Z, Kharazmi A, Wu H, Faber V, Moser C, Krogh HK, Rygaard J, Hoiby N. (1998). Effects of ginseng treatment on neutrophil chemiluminescence and immunoglobulin G subclasses in a rat model of chronic *Pseudomonas aeruginosa* pneumonia. *Clinical Diagnostics and Laboratory Immunology* 5(6):882-887.

Sonnerborg A, Saaf J, Alexius B, Strannegard O, Wahlund LO, Wetterberg L. (1990). Quantitative detection of brain aberrations in human immunodeficiency virus type 1-infected individuals by magnetic resonance imaging. *Journal of Infectious Diseases* 162(6):1245-1251.

Sorenson WG. (1999). Fungal spores: Hazardous to health? *Environmental Health Perspectives* 3:469-472.

St. George IM. (1996). Did Cook's sailors have Tapanui flu? Chronic fatigue syndrome on the resolution. *New Zealand Medical Journal* 109(1014):15-17.

Steinberg P, McNutt BE, Marshall P, Schenck C, Lurie N, Pheley A, Peterson PK. (1996). Double-blind placebo-controlled study of the efficacy of oral terfenadine in the treatment of chronic fatigue syndrome. *Journal of Allergy and Clinical Immunology* 97(1 Pt. 1):119-126.

Steinberg P, Pheley A, Peterson PK. (1996). Influence of immediate hypersensitivity skin reaction on delayed reactions in patients with chronic fatigue syndrome. *Journal of Allergy and Clinical Immunology* 98(6 Pt. 1):1126-1128.

Sterzl I, Zamrazil V. (1996). Endocrinopathy in the differential diagnosis of chronic fatigue syndrome, *Vnitrni Lekarstvi* 42(9):624-626.

Stitz L, Bilzer T, Tich JA, Rott R. (1993). Pathogenesis of Borna disease. *Archives of Virology* 7:135-151.

Stone AA, Broderick JE, Porter LS, Kaell AT. (1997). The experience of rheumatoid arthritis pain and fatigue: Examining momentary reports and correlates over one week. *Arthritis Care and Research* 10(3):185-193.

Straus SE. (1990). Intravenous immunoglobulin treatment for the chronic fatigue syndrome. *American Journal of Medicine* 89:551-553.

Straus SE, Dale JK, Peter JB, Dinarello CA. (1989). Circulating lymphokine levels in the chronic fatigue syndrome. *Journal of Infectious Diseases* 160(6):1085-1086.

Straus SE, Tosato G, Armstrong G, Lawley T, Preble OT, Henle W, Davey R, Pearson G, Epstein J, Brus I, et al. (1985). Persisting illness and fatigue in adults with evidence of Epstein-Barr virus infection. *Annals of Internal Medicine* 102(1):7-16.

Strickland P, Morriss R, Wearden A, Deakin B. (1998). A comparison of salivary cortisol in chronic fatigue syndrome, community depression and healthy controls. *Journal of Affective Disorders* 47(1-3):191-194.

Subira ML, Castilla A, Civeira MP, Prieto J. (1989). Deficient display of CD3 on lymphocytes of patients with chronic fatigue syndrome. *Journal of Infectious Diseases* 160(1):165-166.

Suzuki T, Suzuki N, Daynes RA, Engleman EG. (1991). Dehydroepiandrosterone enhances IL2 production and cytotoxic effector function of human T cells. *Clinical Immunology and Immunopathology* 61(2):202-211.

Swanink CM, Stolk-Engelaar VM, van der Meer JW, Vercoulen JH, Bleijenberg G, Fennis, JM, Galama JM, Hoogkamp-Korstanje JA. (1998). *Yersinia enterocolitica* and the chronic fatigue syndrome. *Journal of Infection* 36(3):269-272.

Swanink CM, Vercoulen JH, Galama JM, Roos MT, Meyaard L, van der Ven-Jongekrijg J, de Nijs R, Bleijenberg G, Fennis JF, Miedema F, van der Meer JW. (1996). Lymphocyte subsets, apoptosis, and cytokines in patients with chronic fatigue syndrome. *Journal of Infectious Diseases* 173(2):460-463.

Takao T, Hashimoto K, De Souza EB. (1995). Modulation of interleukin-1 receptors in the brain-endocrine-immune axis by stress and infection. *Brain, Behavior and Immunity* 9:276.

Takao T, Nagano I, Tojo C, Takemura T, Makino S, Hashimoto K, De Souza EB. (1996). Age-related reciprocal modulation of interleukin-1beta and interleukin-1 receptors in the mouse brain-endocrine-immune axis. *Neuroimmunomodulation* 3:205.

Talal N, Dauphinée MJ, Dang H, Alexander SS, Hart DJ, Garry RF. (1990). Detection of serum antibodies to retroviral proteins in patients with primary Sjogren's syndrome (autoimmune exocrinopathy). *Arthritis and Rheumatism* 33(6):774-781.

Talal N, Garry RF, Schur PH, Alexander S, Dauphinee MJ, Livas IH, Ballester A, Takei M, Dang H. (1990). A conserved idiotype and antibodies to retroviral proteins in systemic lupus erythematosus. *Journal of Clinical Investigation* 85(6):1866-1887.

Tarbleton P. (1995). To Whom It May Concern. *Affidavit to the SA Medical Council.* January.

Targan S, Stebbing N. (1982). In vitro interactions of purified cloned human interferons on NK cells: Enhanced activation. *Journal of Immunology* 129:934-935.

Tedla N, Dwyer J, Truskett P, Taub D, Wakefield D, Lloyd A. (1999). Phenotypic and functional characterization of lymphocytes derived from normal and HIV-1-infected human lymph nodes. *Clinical and Experimental Immunology* 117(1):92-99.

Teitelbaum JE, Bird B, Weiss A, Gould L. (1999). Low-dose hydrocortisone for chronic fatigue syndrome. *Journal of the American Medical Association* 281(20):1887-1888.

Tian J, Lehmann PV, Kaufman DL. (1994). T cell cross-reactivity between coxsackievirus and glutamate decarboxylase is associated with a murine diabetes susceptibility allele. *Journal of Experimental Medicine* 180:1979-1984.

Tirelli U, Marotta G, Improta S, Pinto A. (1994). Immunological abnormalities in patients with chronic fatigue syndrome. *Scandinavian Journal of Immunology* 40(6):601-608.

Tobach et al. (1956). *American Journal of Physiology* 187:399-402.

Tobi M, Morag A, Ravid Z, Chowers I, Feldman-Weiss V, Michaeli Y, Ben-Chetrit E, Shalit M, Knobler H. (1982). Prolonged atypical illness associated with serological evidence of persistent Epstein-Barr infection. *Lancet* 1(8263):61-64.

Tosato G, Straus S, Henle W, Pike SE, Blaese RM. (1985). Characteristic T cell dysfunction in patients with chronic active Epstein-Barr virus infection (chronic infectious mononucleosis). *Journal of Immunology* 134(5):3082-3088.

Treib J, Grauer MT, Haas A, Langenbach J, Holzer G, Woessner R. (2000). Chronic fatigue syndrome in patients with Lyme borreliosis. *European Journal of Neurology* 43(2):107-109.

Trujillo JR, McLane MF, Lee T-H, Essex M. (1993). Molecular mimicry between the human immunodeficiency virus type 1 gp120 V3 loop and human brain proteins. *Journal of Virology* 67:7711-7715.

Tsudo M, Ichiyama T, Uchino H. (1984). Expression of Tac antigen on activated normal human B cells. *Journal of Experimental Medicine* 160:612-617.

Turnbull A, Rivier C. (1995a). Brain-periphery connections: Do they play a role in mediating the effect of centrally injected interleukin-1 beta on gonadal function? *Neuroimmunomodulation* 2:224.

Turnbull AV, Rivier C. (1995b). Regulation of the HPA axis by cytokines. *Brain, Behavior and Immunity* 9:153.

Uter W. (2000). Chronic fatigue syndrome and nickel allergy. *Contact Dermatitis* 42(1):56-57.

van der Meer MJ, Hermus AR, Pesman GJ, Sweep CG. (1996). Effects of cytokines on pituitary beta-endorphin and adrenal corticosterone release in vitro. *Cytokine* 8:238.

van der Meer MJ, Sweep CG, Pesman GJ, Tilders F J, Hermus AR. (1996). Chronic stimulation of the hypothalamus-pituitary-adrenal axis in rats by interleukin 1beta: Central and peripheral mechanisms. *Cytokine* 8:910.

Van Eldik LJ, Zimmer DB. (1987). Secretion of S-100 from rat C6 glioma cells. *Brain Research* 436:367-370.

Van Snick J. (1990). Interleukin-6: An overview. *Annual Reviews in Immunology* 8:253-278.

Vara-Thorbeck R, Guerrero JA, Ruiz-Requena E, Garcia-Carriazo M. (1996). Can the use of growth hormone reduce the postoperative fatigue syndrome? *World Journal of Surgery* 20(1):81-86; discussion 86-87.

Vasina IG, Frolov EP, Serebriakov NG. (1975). Sympathico-adrenal system activity in a primary immune response. *Zhurnal Mikrobiologii, Epidemiologii i Imunobiologii* 10(9):88-92.

Villemain F, Chatenoud L, Galinowski A, Homo-Delarche F, Ginestet D, Loo H, Zarifian E, Bach JF. (1989). Aberrant T cell-mediated immunity in untreated schizophrenic patients: Deficient interleukin-2 production. *American Journal of Psychiatry* 146(5):609-616.

Visser J, Blauw B, Hinloopen B, Brommer E, de Kloet ER, Kluft C, Nagelkerken L. (1998). CD4 T lymphocytes from patients with chronic fatigue syndrome have decreased interferon-gamma production and increased sensitivity to dexamethasone. *Journal of Infectious Diseases* 177(2):451-454.

Vitkovic L, Chatham JJ, da Cunha A. (1995). Distinct expressions of three cytokines by IL-1-stimulated astrocytes in vitro and in AIDS brain. *Brain, Behavior and Immunity* 9:378.

Vojdani A, Choppa PC, Tagle C, Andrin R, Samimi B, Lapp CW. (1998). Detection of *Mycoplasma* genus and *Mycoplasma fermentans* by PCR in patients with chronic fatigue syndrome. *FEMS Immunology and Medical Microbiology* 22: 355-365.

Vojdani A, Franco AR. (1999). Multiplex PCR for the detection of *Mycoplasma fermentans, M. hominis* and *M. penetrans* in patients with chronic fatigue syndrome, fibromyalgia, rheumatoid arthritis and Gulf War illness. *Journal of Chronic Fatigue Syndrome* 5:187-197.

Vojdani A, Ghoneum M, Choppa PC, Magtoto L, Lapp CW. (1997). Elevated apoptotic cell population in patients with chronic fatigue syndrome: The pivotal role of protein kinase RNA. *Journal of Internal Medicine* 242(6):465-478.

Vojdani A, Lapp CW. (1999). Interferon-induced proteins are elevated in blood samples of patients with chemically or virally induced chronic fatigue syndrome. *Immunopharmacology and Immunotoxicology* 21(2):175-202.

Vollmer-Conna U, Hickie I, Hadzi-Pavlovic D, Tymms K, Wakefield D, Dwyer J, Lloyd A. (1997). Intravenous immunoglobulin is ineffective in the treatment of patients with chronic fatigue syndrome. *American Journal of Medicine* 103(1):38-43.

Vollmer-Conna U, Lloyd A, Hickie I, Wakefield D. (1998). Chronic fatigue syndrome: An immunological perspective. *Australian and New Zealand Journal of Psychiatry* 32(4):523-527.

von Mikecz A, Konstantinov K, Buchwald DS, Gerace L, Tan EM. (1997). High frequency of autoantibodies in patients with chronic fatigue syndrome. *Arthritis and Rheumatism* 40(2):295-305.

Wakefield D, Lloyd A, Brockman A. (1990). Immunoglobulin subclass abnormalities in patients with chronic fatigue syndrome. *Journal of Pediatric Infectious Diseases* 9(8):S50-S53.

Wallace HL II, Natelson B, Gause W, Hay J. (1999). Human herpesviruses in chronic fatigue syndrome. *Journal of Clinical Diagnostic and Laboratory Immunology* 6(2):216-223.

Wang B, Gladman DD, Urowitz MB. (1998). Fatigue in lupus is not correlated with disease activity. *Journal of Rheumatology* 25(5):892-895.

Watanobe H, Anzai J, Nigawara T, Habu S, Takebe, K. (1996). Effects of gender and gonadectomy on ACTH response to interleukin-1beta in the rat: Comparison with the modulation of ACTH response to immobilization stress. *Neuroimmunomodulation* 3:254.

Watanobe H, Nasushita R, Takebe K. (1995). A study on the role of circulating prostaglandin E2 in the adrenocorticotropin response to intravenous administration of interleukin-1 beta in the rat. *Neuroendocrinology* 62:596.

Watson J, Mochizuki D. (1980). Interleukin-2: A class of T cell growth factor. *Immunological Reviews* 51:257-278.

Weinstein L. (1987). Thyroiditis and "chronic infectious mononucleosis." *New England Journal of Medicine* 317:1225-1226.

Weiss JM, Quan N, Sundar SK. (1994). Widespread activation and consequences of interleukin-1 in the brain. *Annals of the New York Academy of Sciences* 741:338-357.

Westemann J, Pabst R. (1996). How organ specific is the migration of "naïve" and "memory" T cells? *Immunology Today* 17:278-282.

White PD, Thomas JM, Amess J, Crawford DH, Grover SA, Kangro HO, Clare AW. (1998). Incidence, risk and prognosis of acute and chronic fatigue syndromes and psychiatric disorders after glandular fever. *British Journal of Psychiatry* 173:475-481.

Whiteside TL. (1994). Cytokine measurements and interpretation in human disease. *Journal of Clinical Immunology* 14:327-339.

Whiteside TL, Friberg D. (1998). Natural killer cells and natural killer cell activity in chronic fatigue syndrome. *American Journal of Medicine* 105(3A):27S-34S.

Wilt SG, Milward E, Zhou JM, Nagasato K, Patton H, Rusten R, Griffin DE, O'Connor M, Dubois-Dalag M. (1995). In vitro evidence for a dual role of tumor necrosis factor in human immunodeficiency virus type 1 encephalopathy. *Annals of Neurology* 37(3):381-394.

Woldehiwe T. (1991). Lymphomatic subpopulations in peripheral blood of sheep experimentally infected with tick-borne disease. *Research Veterinary Scientist.* July.

Wolfe F, Hawley DJ, Wilson K. (1996). The prevalence and meaning of fatigue in rheumatic disease. *Journal of Rheumatology* 23(8):1407-1417.

Wong HCG. (1999). Probable false authentication of herbal plants: Ginseng. *Archives of Internal Medicine* 159:1142.

Wood B, Wessely S, Papadopoulos A, Poon L, Checkley S. (1998). Salivary cortisol profiles in chronic fatigue syndrome. *Neuropsychobiology* 37(1):1-4.

Wood TL, O'Donnell SL, Levison SW. (1995). Cytokines regulate IGF binding proteins in the CNS. *Progress in Growth Factor Research* 6:181.

Wu CY, Sarfati M, Heusser C, Fournier S, Rubio-Trujillo M, Peleman R, Delespesse G. (1991). Glucocorticoids increase the synthesis of immunoglobulin E by interleukin 4-stimulated human lymphocytes. *Journal of Clinical Investigation* 87(3):870-877.

Yamaguchi K, Sawada T, Naraki T, Igata-Yi R, Shiraki H, Horii Y, Ishii T, Ikeda K, Asou N, Okabe H, Mochizuki M, Takahashi K, Yamada S, Kubo K, Yashiki S, Waltrip RW II, Carbone KM. (1999). Detection of Borna disease virus-reactive antibodies from patients with psychiatric disorders and from horses by electrochemiluminescence immunoassay. *Clinical Diagnostic and Laboratory Immunology* 6(5):696-700.

Young AH, Sharpe M, Clements A, Dowling B, Hawton KE, Cowen PJ. (1998). Basal activity of the hypothalamic-pituitary-adrenal axis in patients with the chronic fatigue syndrome (naurasthenia). *Biological Psychiatry* 43(3):236-237.

Zlotnik A, Shimonkewitz P, Gefter ML, Kappler J, Marrack P. (1983). Characterization of the gamma interferon-mediated induction of antigen-presenting ability in P388D cells. *Journal of Immunology* 131(6):2814-2820.

Zwilling BS, Lafuse WP, Brown D, Pearl D. (1992). Characterization of ACTH-mediated suppression of MHC class II expression by murine peritoneal macrophages. *Journal of Neuroimmunology* 39(1-2):133-138.

Index

ß2-adrenoreceptor-cAMP-protein
      kinase A pathway, 7
17-alpha-hydroxyprogesterone, 16

Ablashi, DV, 50
Acquired immunodeficiency syndrome
      (AIDS), 3, 44, 73
   dementia complex, 13, 45
ACTH, 10, 11, 16
   -releasing factor, 37
Active disease, 58
Acute fatigue syndrome, 50
Acute febrile illness, 18
ADCC, 32, 77
Adrenocorticotropin hormone (ACTH),
      10, 11, 16
   -releasing factor, 37
AIDS, 3, 44, 73
   dementia complex, 13, 45
Allergic reactions, 3, 18, 33, 42
Alpha-melanocyte-stimulating
      hormone, 8, 65
Alzheimer's disease, 13, 38
Anabolic steroids, 12
Ankylosing spondylitis, 58
Anorexia, 18
Antibody-dependent cellular
      cytotoxicity (ADCC), 32, 77
Antigen-presenting cells (A.C.), 71
Antigliadin, 47, 57
Antinuclear antibodies (AA), 47, 57
Anti-p80 coilin antibodies, 47, 57
Anti–smooth-muscle antibodies, 57
Antithyroid antibodies, 57
Apoptosis, 28-29
Appetite loss, 39
Arthralgia, 54
Arthus reaction, depressed, 8
Asthma, 3, 18, 66, 67
Astrocytes, 36
Astrocytosis, reactive, 13
Autoantibodies, 46-47

Autoantibody production, 43
Autoimmune disease, 24, 40, 59
Autoimmune fatigue syndrome,
      children and, 58
Autoimmunity
   B cells and, 26
   and CFS, 56-59
   IL-4 and, 42
   IL-6 and, 43
Autologous reinfusion, lymph node
      cells, 4

B cells, 1, 46
B lymphocytes, 26, 27-29, 69
Bacillus Camelet-Guerin (BCG), 68
Bacteria, CFS and, 54-56
Baraniuk, JN, 33
Barker, E, 25, 26, 27, 32
Baschetti, R, 18
Bax gene, 28
Bcl-2 gene, 28
Bell's palsy, 54
Bennett, AL, 43
Beta-2 microglobulin, 44
Bloodborne cytokines, 12
Borish, L, 33
Borna disease virus (BDV), 53
Borok, G, 33
Borrelia, 54
Borrelia burgdorferi, 55
Borrelia duttoni, 55
Borysiewicz, LK, 23, 30
Bounous, G, 27, 28
Brain dopamine, replacement of
      depleted, 19
Buchwald, D
   and C-reactive protein, 47
   and IL-6, 42
   and immune cells, 21, 23
   and natural killer cells, 30
   and neopterin, 44, 45
Buspirone, 19

C1q binding, 47
Caligiuri, M, 26
Cancer, 29, 44, 74, 76
Catabolism, 18
Catecholamine neurotransmitter levels, 8
CD3, 27
CD4, 2, 22-25, 42
CD4/CD8 ratio, 22
CD4+CD45RA+ lymphocyte subset, depletion of, 46
CD45RA+, 59
CD45RO+, 59
CD5, 26
CD8, 2, 22-25
CD26, 24
Cell therapy, 79
Cellular function, poor, 61-62
Cellular toxicity, antibody-dependent, 26
Central nervous system (CNS)
microglia, 35
trauma to, 14, 16
Cerebrospinal fluid (CSF), 13
CFS. *See* Chronic fatigue syndrome
Chao, CC, 42, 43
Cheney, PR, 40
Chlamydia, 54
Chronic fatigue syndrome (CFS), 4
and immune abnormalities, significance of, 21
infectious agents as cause of, 49-56
signs/symptoms of, 37, 61. *See also* Fatigue; Fever
sudden onset of, 61
Chronic progressive (CP) types, 43
Ciliary neurotrophic factor (CNTF), 14
Circulating immune complexes, 47
Cleare, AJ, 17-18
CNS
microglia, 35
trauma to, 14, 16
Cognitive difficulty, increased, 28
Cognitive difficulty scale (CDS), 44
Cohen, S, 62
Cold agglutinins, 47, 57
Complement, depressed levels of, 47
Concanavalin A, 9
Conti, F, 32

Corpora lutea-induced prolactin (PRL) release, 12
Corticosterone, 10
Corticotropin-releasing factor, stimulation of, 8, 65
Corticotropin-releasing hormone (CRH), 10, 16
Cortisol, 16, 17, 37, 66
Corynebacterium parvum, 35
Coxiella burnetti, 56
C-reactive protein, 47
CRH, 10, 16
Cross-talk, nervous and immune systems and, 7
Cryoglobulins, 47, 57
Cytokines, 1, 9, 12, 35, 36-45

Davis, JM, 41
De Becker, P, 16
De novo synthesis, 39
Dehydroepiandrosterone (DHEA), 16, 65-66
Delayed-type hypersensitivity (DTH), 33, 66
Demyelination, 39
Depression
and autoimmunity, 58
and borna disease virus, 53
and IFNs, 41
and NK cell activity, 8-9
and stress, 67
and TGF-beta, 43
Dermal dendritic cells, 36
Dermatomyositis, 58
Desmopressin (DDAVP), 17
Dexamethasone (DEX), 42
DHEA, 16, 65-66
DHEA-sulphate (DHEA-S), 16
Dilated cardiomyopathy, 50
Diptheria, tetanus, and pertussis (DP) vaccine, 64
Distress, increase in, 62-63
Diurnal change, decreased, 16
DTH, 33, 66

E type immunoglobulin bullets, 3
EBV. *See* Epstein-Barr virus
Eczema, 66, 67

Electroencephalogram slow-wave
  activity, 19
Elenkov, IJ, 7
Endocrine disease, immune-mediated, 41
Endogenous catecholamines, 7
Endothelial cells, 36, 38
Endotoxin, 10
Eosinophil cationic protein (ECP), 32
Eosinophils, 32-33
Epinephrine, 7
Epstein-Barr virus (EBV)
  and autoimmunity, 58, 59
  and herpesvirus, 50
  and immunoglobulins, 46
  and NK cells, 30
  and stress, 66
  and T lymphocytes, 24
Erythema migrans, 54
Ether-laparatomy stress, 10

Facial pain, 15
Fatigue
  and autoimmunity, 58
  borrelia and, 54
  herpesvirus and, 50
  and IFN-alpha therapy, 41
  and mRNA expression, 35
  and neuroendocrinology, 15, 18
  postdialysis, 39
  ross river virus and, 53
  and T lymphocyctes, 25
Fever, 2, 18, 31
Fibroblasts, 36
Fibromyalgia, 58, 79
Fidia Farmaceutici Italiani Deriviate
  Industriali e Affini, 76
Fletcher, MA, 59, 71
Fluctuation, clinical manifestation, 23
Folacin, 75
Follicle-stimulating hormone (FSH), 11
Follicular stage, menstruation, 38
Food intolerance, 33
Franco, E, 24
Fungi, CFS and, 56

G2/M boundary, 28-29
Gastric tumor, 77

Gastrointestinal inflammatory disease,
  19
Ginseng, 77
Glandular fever, 50
Glucocorticoids, 9-10
Gluconutrient compound, 29, 31
Glutathione (GSH), 27-28
Gold, D, 29
Gottfries, C-G, 75
Growth factors, 7, 14, 65
Growth hormone, 37
Gulf War syndrome, 64-65, 79
Gulick, T, 38
Gupta, S
  and B lymphocytes, 26, 27
  and IL-10, 43
  and monocytes, 32
  and T lymphocytes, 23, 27
  and TNFs, 39

Hassan, IS, 25, 27, 28
Headaches, 25, 78
Helper-induced cells, 22-25
Hematological malignancy, 40
Hemophilus influenzae, 13
Hepatitis B, 76, 77
Herbal medicine, 5
Herpesvirus, 50-51, 59, 62
High-titer measles vaccine, 64
HHV-6, 50, 51
HHV-7, 51
HIV-1-associated disease, 21
HLA-DQ3 marker, 46, 57
HLA-DR marker, 24, 25, 32
Homeostasis, threats to, 9
Hormonal secretions, induction of, 8
Hormones, 35
  decreased levels of, 18
HPA axis. *See* Hypothalamic-pituitary-
  adrenal (HPA) axis
Hudson, M, 17
Human herpesvirus-6 (HHV-6), 50, 51
Human leukocyte antigen (HLA)
  molecules, 4, 24
Humoral immunity, 2, 8
Hydrocortisone treatment, 20
Hypegammaglogulinemia, 43
Hypersensitivity, delayed-type, 33

Hypoglycemia, reduced GH response
    to, 17
Hypotension, 38
Hypothalamic feedback loop, 37
Hypothalamic-pituitary-adrenal (HPA)
    axis
    defects in, 18, 19
    the nervous system and, 7, 8, 9
    neuroendocrinology and, 15, 17
    -related hormonal deficiency, 41
    and stress-mediated change, 65, 66
Hypothalamus, 2, 37
Hypothyroidism, 41

IFN-gamma, 14, 41
IgA levels, 46
IGF-binding proteins (IGFBPs), 14, 17
IGFs, 14, 17
IgG antibody, 52
IgG levels, 46, 62
IgM antibody, 52
IL-1, 2, 8, 36-39
IL-1 receptor antagonist (IL-1Ra), 9, 12
IL-1alpha, 10, 36
IL-1beta, 9, 10, 11, 12, 13-14, 36
IL-1Ra, 9, 12
IL-2, 3, 5, 10, 40, 59
IL-2 receptor (CD25), 24
IL-4, 28, 42, 69
Il-5, 28
IL-6, 10, 28, 42-43
IL-10, 43
Illness burden scores, 39
Immune activation, 61
Immunizations, childhood, 71. *See also*
    Vaccinations
Immunodysregulation, 78
Immunoglobulation, 62
Immunoglobulin bullets, E type, 3
Immunoglobulin replacement therapy,
    46
Immunoglobulin synthesis, 28, 45
Immunoglobulins, 45-46, 71
Immunotherapy, 5
    lymph node cell-based, 71-73
Incline, Nevada, 55
Indoleamine 2,3-dioxygenase, 44
Inducible NO synthase (iNOS), 31
Infection, and sudden onset of CFS, 61

Infectious agents, as cause of CFS,
    49-56
Influenza vaccine, 4
iNos, 19
Insecticides, exposure to, 67
Insulin-like growth factors (IGFs), 14,
    17
Interferon (IFN)-gamma, 7, 30
Interferons (IFNs), 40-41
Interleukin-1 (IL-1), 2, 8, 36-39
Interleukin-2 (IL-2), 3, 5, 10, 40, 59
Interleukin-4 (IL-4), 42, 69
Interleukin-6 (IL-6), 10, 28, 42-43
Interleukin-8 (IL-8), 8
Interleuking-10 (IL-10), 43
Interleukin-12 (IL-12), 3, 7
Intracerebroventricular (ICV) injection,
    11
Isapirone, 17
Itoh, Y, 57

Japan
    BDV in, 53
    Kaken Pharmaceutical Co., Ltd., 76
    and tuberculin skin-tests, 68
Jenner, and vaccination, 70
Jones, J, 22
Juvenile (type 1) diabetes, 50

K562 cells, 29
Kaken Pharmaceutical Co., Ltd.
    (Japan), 76
Kaposi's sarcoma, 73
Karnofsky score, 72
Kavelaars, A, 14-15
Keller, RH, 46
Kibler, R, 30
Klimas, N
    and autoimmunity, 59
    and B lymphocytes, 26
    and immunoglobulins, 46
    and lymph node study, University of
        Miami, 71
    and NK cells, 30
    and T lymphocytes, 23
Konstantinov, K, 46
Kynurenic acid, 45

LaManca, JJ, 18
Lamin B1, 57
Landay, AL, 23, 25, 26
Large joint arthritis, 54
L-Arginine (L-Arg), 30
Lentivirus, 52
Leukocyte 2'5'-oligoadenylate
    synthetase, 30
Levine, PH, 29
Lewis rats, 37
Leydig cell function, 12
LH, 11, 37
Linde, A, 37, 40, 41, 44, 45
L-kynurenine, 44
Lloyd, AR, 23, 26, 37, 39
Low NK syndrome (LNKS), 31-32
L-tryptophan, 44
Lung tumor, 77
Lusso, P, 30
Luteal stage, menstruation, 38
Luteinizing hormone (LH), 11, 37
Lutgendorf, S, 28
Lyme borreliosis, 54
Lyme disease, 54, 55
Lymph node cells, 59
    autologous reinfusion of, 4
    CD3+, 24
    ex vivo activation of, 36
    immunotherapy, 71-73
    as source of serum IL-1alpha, 36
Lymphoid cell, 22
Lymphoproliferative malignancy, 40

M. vaccae, 73-75
Macrophage, 1, 45
Malgach fever, 55
Manic episode, 78
Masuda, A, 26
Mawle, AC, 23, 27, 29, 33
Measles vaccine, 64, 68
Memory loss, 25
"Memory" phenotype, 59
Meningeal fibroblasts, 12
Menstruation, 38
Messenger RNA (mRNA), 36, 42
Methodology, flaws in, 22
Metyrapone, 67
Microbial reactivation, 61
Microglia, 45

"Molecular mimicry," 4, 56
Monoclonal antibodies, 21
Monocytes, 32
Mononucleosis, 37
Morag, A, 30
Morrison, LJ, 26
Moss, RB, 39
mRNA, 36, 42
MS, 8, 43, 50, 59, 65
Multidimensional Fatigue Inventory, 58
Multiple chemical sensitivity, 79
Multiple sclerosis (MS), 8, 43, 50, 59,
    65
Mycobacterium vaccae, 73-75
Mycobacterium vaccae vaccine, 4
Mycoplasma, 54-55
Mycoplasma fermentans, 55
Mycoplasma pneumoniae, 55
Mycoplasmal infection, 55

Nakaya, T, 53
Nasralla, M, 55
Natelson, BH, 23-24, 26, 47
Natural killer (NK) cell, 1, 8, 26, 29-32,
    77
Natural killer cell cytotoxicity (NKCC),
    32, 62, 63
Nausea, 19
Neopterin, 32, 44-45
Neuroborreliosis, 54
Neurocognitive impairment, 54
Neuroendocrinology, 14-20
Neuromodulators, 7, 65
Nueromuscular fatigue, 41
Neuropsychiatric disease, 53
Neurotransmitters, 7, 35, 65
Neutrophilia, exercise-induced, 18, 26
Neutrophils, 26
Nickle allergy, 33, 75
Nightingale, Florence, 55
Nitric oxide (NO), 12, 19, 30
Nitric oxide synthase, induced (iNOS),
    19
NK cell, 1, 8, 26, 29-32, 77
NKCC, 32, 62, 63
Norepinephrine (NE), 7
Nuclear envelope antigens, 46, 57

Ogawa, M, 30
Osteoarthritis, 58
Ovarian function, 11
Oxidative stress, 44

Pall, ML, 19
Panax ginseng, 5, 77-78
Parameters, discrepancy in, 22
Parkinson's disease, 13
Parvovirus B19, 52
Patarca, R
    and IL-2, 40
    and immune cells, 21
    and lymph node study, University of
        Miami, 71
    and neopterin, 44
    and sICAM-1, 45
    and TNFs, 39
PBMCs, 36, 53, 77
Peakman, M, 23, 25, 26, 37, 39
Peripheral blood mononuclear cells
    (PBMCs), 36, 53, 77
PHA, 27, 72, 77
Phagocytosis index, deficit of, 32
Phenelzine sulfate, 78
Phytohemagglutinin (PHA), 27, 72, 77
Picornavirus, 49
Plaque-forming cell response, 8, 65
Plasma volume, 38
Pokeweek mitogen (PWM), 27
Poliomyelitis, 70
Poliovirus, 45, 70
Poly I-C, 4, 41
Poly (I)-poly (C12U), 36
Polymerase chain reaction, 55
Post viral fatigue syndrome, 1
Postdialysis fatigue, 39
Post-Lyme disease syndrome (PLS), 54
Postpolio fatigue, 19
Postpolio syndrome, 41, 50
Post–Q-fever fatigue syndrome (QFS),
        43, 55-56
Premenstruation, 38
Prieto, J, 32
Procainamide-induced lupus, 59
Proinflammatory cytokines, 36-41
Prolactin, 37
Prolactin secretion, increased, 19
Pro-opiomelanocortin, 8

Prostaglandins (PG), 10, 38
Protein kinase RNA (PKR), 29
Pseudomonas aeruginosa, 77
Psychiatric trauma, and sudden onset of
        CFS, 61
Psychosocial stressors, 62
Pyrogens, 2

Q-fever, 55
    post-, 43, 56
Quality of Life (QOL), survey, 31
Quinolinic acid (QUIN), 45

Raji cell, 47
Rasmussen, AK, 37, 39, 40, 47
Reaction allergen-specific testing
        (RAST), 32-33
Regland, B, 75
Relapse/remitting (R/R), 43
Respiratory infection, 50, 62
Retrovirus, 52
Reverse transcriptase-coupled
        polymerase chain reaction
        (RT-PCR), 36, 53
Rh status, 27
Rheumatic autoimmune disease, 46, 57
Rheumatoid arthritis, 3, 19, 58, 59
Rheumatoid factor, 47, 57
Rhinovirus, 62
Rickettsiae, 55-56
Roberts, TK, 27
Rocky Mountain spotted fever, 55
Rook, GA, 64, 73, 74
Ross river virus, 52-53
RT-PCR, 36, 53
Rubella vaccine, 4

S phase, 28
Salivary cortisol, 17
Sandman, CA, 23
Sauton, and *M. vaccae*, 74
sCD120a, 40
sCD120b, 40
Schizophrenia, 53
Schutzer, SE, 54
Scott, LV, 16, 17

See, DM, 29, 31
Sepsis syndrome, 21
Serum neopterin, 39
Shared hormones, 7, 65
Short Form-36 health questionnaire
(SF-36), 25
Sick building syndrome, 79
Sickness Impact Profile (SIP), 25, 63
sIL-2R, 40
sIL-6R, 43
SIP Physical Impairment, 25, 28
Sizofiran, 76-77
Sjoegren's syndrome, 58, 59
SLE, 3, 43, 58, 59
Sleep abnormalities, 17, 58
Slow-wave sleep, 37
Smallpox, 70
Smoking, 75
Smooth-muscle cells, 38
anti-, 47, 57
S-nitroso-N-acetylpenicillamine, 31
Soluble antigens, response to, 27
Soluble CD8 (sCD8), 45
Soluble ICAM-1 (sICAM-1), 45
Soluble IL-2 receptor, 40
Soluble IL-6 receptor, 42
Soluble receptor, 36-39
Soluble TNF-receptor (sTNF-R),
12-13, 39-40
Soluble TNF-receptor type I (sTNF-
RI), 40, 72
Somnolence, 2
Staphylococcus vaccine, 4, 75-76
Stealth virus, 51-52
sTNF-R, 12-13, 39-40
sTNF-RI, 40, 72
sTNF-RII, 40
Straus, SE, 22, 30, 41
Stress, 8, 10, 15
Stressors, 58
Hurricane Andrew as, 63
Subcortical lesions, 45
Surface-marker phenotyping, 22
Swanink, CM, 24, 25, 29, 38
Sympathetic nervous system, 7, 8
Sympathetic/noradrenergic innervation,
7
Symptom Impact Profile, 72
Syphilis, false serological positivity for,
47, 57

Systemic lupus erythematosus (SLE),
3, 43, 58, 59
Systemic unique hormones, 7

T cells
activation of, 1
receptors, 2
T lymphocytes, 22-25, 27-29. *See also*
T cells
T-cell growth factor, 30
Tedla, N, 59
Testicular function, 12
Thalidomide, 13
T-helper cells, 2
T-helper type 1 (TH1), 2, 3, 4, 5, 8
T-helper type 2 (TH2), 2, 3, 4, 5, 8, 63
Therapeutic intervention, 4-5
TH1, 2, 3, 4, 5, 8
TH1 cytokines, 36-39
TH1/TH2 paradigm, 3
balance modulation, 69-78
imbalance, 61-68
TH2, 2, 3, 4, 5, 8, 63
TH2 cytokines, 42-43
Thyrotropin, 37
Tirelli, U, 26
Tissue macrophage, 36
TNF. *See* Tumor necrosis factor
TNF-alpha, 10, 39
TNF-beta, 39
Toxins, exposure to, 61
Treib, J, 54
Tremulousness, 78
T-suppressor cells, 2
Tuberculosis, 67
Tumor growth, 8, 65
Tumor growth factor-beta (TGF-beta),
43
Tumor necrosis factor (TNF), 2, 37,
39-40
-alpha, 7, 8
Type 1/proinflammatory cytokines, 7

Upper-respiratory tract infections
(URIs), 50, 62
Urinary cortisol, 17, 18
Urinary free cortisol (UFC), 15

Vaccinations, 63-64, 67-68
Vaccine, 79
Vasodilators, 38
Verbal memory, decrease in, 41
Vimentin, deficit of, 32
Viral infection, 40, 70
Viruses, CFS and, 49-50, 70
Visser, J, 42
Vitamin B$_{12}$, 75
Vojdani, A, 28, 41

Vollmer-Conna, U, 35
von Mikecz, A, 46

Wallace II, HL, 51

Yersinia, 56
Yersinia outer membrane proteins
      (YOPs), 56

AAO-9557